FINANCING VACCINES
IN THE 21ST CENTURY

Assuring Access and Availability

Committee on the Evaluation of Vaccine Purchase Financing
in the United States
Board on Health Care Services

INSTITUTE OF MEDICINE
OF THE NATIONAL ACADEMIES

THE NATIONAL ACADEMIES PRESS
Washington, D.C.
www.nap.edu

THE NATIONAL ACADEMIES PRESS   500 Fifth Street, N.W.   Washington, DC 20001

NOTICE: The project that is the subject of this report was approved by the Governing Board of the National Research Council, whose members are drawn from the councils of the National Academy of Sciences, the National Academy of Engineering, and the Institute of Medicine. The members of the committee responsible for the report were chosen for their special competences and with regard for appropriate balance.

Support for this project was provided by the Centers of Disease Control and Prevention. The views presented in this report are those of the Institute of Medicine Committee on the Evaluation of Vaccine Purchase Financing in the United States and are not necessarily those of the funding agencies.

Library of Congress Cataloging-in-Publication Data

Financing vaccines in the 21st century : assuring access and availability / Committee on the Evaluation of Vaccine Purchase Financing in the United States, Board on Health Care Services.
    p. ; cm.
Includes bibliographical references.
  ISBN 0-309-08979-4 (pbk.)—ISBN 0-309-52619-1 (PDF)
  1. Vaccination—United States—Planning. 2. Vaccines—Economic aspects—United States. 3. Vaccination—Economic aspects—United States. 4. Vaccination—Government policy—United States.
  [DNLM: 1. Mass Immunization—economics—United States. 2. Vaccines—economics—United States. WA 110 F4818 2003] I. Title: Financing vaccines in the twenty-first century. II. Institute of Medicine (U.S.). Committee on the Evaluation of Vaccine Purchase Financing in the United States.
  RA638.F54 2003
  614.4'7—dc22   2003018817

Additional copies of this report are available from the National Academies Press, 500 Fifth Street, N.W., Lockbox 285, Washington, DC 20055; (800) 624-6242 or (202) 334-3313 (in the Washington metropolitan area); Internet, http://www.nap.edu.

For more information about the Institute of Medicine, visit the IOM home page at: **www.iom.edu.**

"Knowing is not enough; we must apply.
Willing is not enough; we must do."

—Goethe

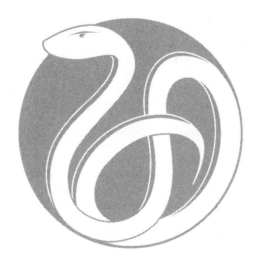

INSTITUTE OF MEDICINE
OF THE NATIONAL ACADEMIES

Shaping the Future for Health

THE NATIONAL ACADEMIES
Advisers to the Nation on Science, Engineering, and Medicine

The **National Academy of Sciences** is a private, nonprofit, self-perpetuating society of distinguished scholars engaged in scientific and engineering research, dedicated to the furtherance of science and technology and to their use for the general welfare. Upon the authority of the charter granted to it by the Congress in 1863, the Academy has a mandate that requires it to advise the federal government on scientific and technical matters. Dr. Bruce M. Alberts is president of the National Academy of Sciences.

The **National Academy of Engineering** was established in 1964, under the charter of the National Academy of Sciences, as a parallel organization of outstanding engineers. It is autonomous in its administration and in the selection of its members, sharing with the National Academy of Sciences the responsibility for advising the federal government. The National Academy of Engineering also sponsors engineering programs aimed at meeting national needs, encourages education and research, and recognizes the superior achievements of engineers. Dr. Wm. A. Wulf is president of the National Academy of Engineering.

The **Institute of Medicine** was established in 1970 by the National Academy of Sciences to secure the services of eminent members of appropriate professions in the examination of policy matters pertaining to the health of the public. The Institute acts under the responsibility given to the National Academy of Sciences by its congressional charter to be an adviser to the federal government and, upon its own initiative, to identify issues of medical care, research, and education. Dr. Harvey V. Fineberg is president of the Institute of Medicine.

The **National Research Council** was organized by the National Academy of Sciences in 1916 to associate the broad community of science and technology with the Academy's purposes of furthering knowledge and advising the federal government. Functioning in accordance with general policies determined by the Academy, the Council has become the principal operating agency of both the National Academy of Sciences and the National Academy of Engineering in providing services to the government, the public, and the scientific and engineering communities. The Council is administered jointly by both Academies and the Institute of Medicine. Dr. Bruce M. Alberts and Dr. Wm. A. Wulf are chair and vice chair, respectively, of the National Research Council.

www.national-academies.org

COMMITTEE ON THE EVALUATION OF VACCINE PURCHASE FINANCING IN THE UNITED STATES

FRANK A. SLOAN, Ph.D. (*Chair*), J. Alexander McMahon Professor of Health Policy and Management, and Professor of Economics, Duke University, Durham, North Carolina

STEVE BERMAN, M.D., Professor and Head, Section of General Academic Pediatrics, and Director, Children's Outcomes Research Program, University of Colorado School of Medicine and The Children's Hospital, Denver, Colorado

DAVID CUTLER, Ph.D., Professor, Department of Economics, Harvard University, Cambridge, Massachusetts

ERIC FRANCE, M.D., M.S.P.H., Chief of Preventive Medicine, Kaiser Permanente-Colorado, Denver, Colorado

WILLIAM J. HALL, M.D., Chief, General Medicine/Geriatric Unit, University of Rochester School of Medicine and Dentistry, Rochester, New York

DAVID R. JOHNSON, M.D., M.P.H., Deputy Director and Chief Medical Executive, Michigan Department of Community Health, Lansing, Michigan

ALISON KEITH, Ph.D., Consultant, Health Economist, Pfizer, Inc. (retired), Springdale, Utah

JUNE O'NEILL, Ph.D., Professor of Economics and Finance, Zicklin School of Business, Baruch College, City University of New York, New York, New York

MARK PAULY, Ph.D., Bendheim Professor and Chair, Health Care Systems Department, The Wharton School, University of Pennsylvania, Philadelphia, Pennsylvania

SARA ROSENBAUM, J.D., Hirsh Professor and Chair, Department of Health Policy, George Washington University Medical Center, School of Public Health and Health Services, Washington, D.C.

IRIS R. SHANNON, Ph.D., R.N., Health Consultant and Associate Professor, Health Systems Management, Rush University, Chicago, Illinois

Committee Staff

Rosemary Chalk, Study Director
Robert Giffin, Ph.D., Senior Program Officer
Nakia Johnson, Senior Project Assistant
Ryan Palugod, Senior Project Assistant

Independent Report Reviewers

This report has been reviewed in draft form by individuals chosen for their diverse perspectives and technical expertise, in accordance with procedures approved by the National Research Council's Report Review Committee. The purpose of this independent review is to provide candid and critical comments that will assist the institution in making its published report as sound as possible and to ensure that the report meets institutional standards for objectivity, evidence, and responsiveness to the study charge. The review comments and draft manuscript remain confidential to protect the integrity of the deliberative process. We wish to thank the following individuals for their review of this report:

WILLIAM V. CORR, Executive Vice President, National Center for Tobacco-Free Kids, Washington, DC

HELEN DARLING, M.A., President, Washington Business Group on Health, Washington, DC

SHERRY GLIED, Ph.D., Assistant Professor of Public Health, Columbia University, New York, NY

HENRY G. GRABOWSKI, Ph.D., Professor of Economics and Director of the Program in Pharmaceuticals and Health Economics, Duke University, Durham, NC

RUTH J. KATZ, J.D., M.P.H., Associate Dean of Administration, Yale University, New Haven, CT

TRACY LIEU, M.D., M.P.H., Associate Professor, Department of Ambulatory Care and Prevention, Harvard University, Boston, MA

Contents

EXECUTIVE SUMMARY   1

1   INTRODUCTION   21
    Background, 22
    Conceptual Framework for the Study, 26
    Study Process, 35
    Summing Up, 36
    Organization of the Report, 37

2   ORIGINS AND RATIONALE OF IMMUNIZATION POLICY   39
    Legislative History of Vaccine Policy, 45
    Shared Federal and State Responsibility for Financing, 47
    Shared Public and Private Responsibility for Coverage, 49
    Public and Private Delivery Systems, 51
    Private Vaccine Production, 52
    The Setting of National Vaccine Policy, 56
    Findings, 61

3   PUBLIC AND PRIVATE INSURANCE COVERAGE   63
    Public Insurance Coverage, 66
    Private Insurance Coverage, 69
    Barriers to a Well-Functioning Immunization Finance System, 73
    Findings, 89

4   DELIVERY SYSTEMS   91
     Delivery of Adult and Childhood Vaccines, 91
     The Work of Immunizing, 94
     Provider Reimbursement, 98
     Barriers to a Well-Functioning Immunization Delivery System, 100
     Findings, 105

5   VACCINE SUPPLY   107
     Size and Growth of the Vaccine Market, 107
     Vaccine Production, 109
     Cost Structure, 111
     Research and Development, 116
     Industry Concentration, 121
     Regulation, 126
     Pricing, 127
     Shortages, 131
     Stockpiles, 137
     CDC Contracting, 138
     Barriers to a Well-Functioning Vaccine Supply System, 139
     Findings, 142

6   CONCLUSIONS AND ALTERNATIVE STRATEGIES   145
     Conclusions, 146
     Alternative Strategies, 151
     Weighing the Alternatives, 179

7   RECOMMENDATIONS   183
     Recommendations, 185
     Final Observations, 210

REFERENCES   211

GLOSSARY   221

APPENDICES
A   Recommended Vaccine Schedules (Childhood and Adult)   229
B   List of Contributors   235
C   Survey of State Vaccine Finance Practices   239
D   Overview of Commissioned Papers   241
E   Committee and Staff Biographies   243

Tables, Figures, and Boxes

TABLES

1-1   Change in Annual Morbidity from Vaccine-Preventable Diseases: Prevaccine Baseline and 2002, 24
1-2   Benefit–Cost Ratios for Selected Vaccines, 28
1-3   Prices of Selected U.S. Vaccines: 1980 Versus 2003, 29
1-4   Vaccines for Children Program: CDC Vaccine Price List, 30

2-1   Government Roles in Immunization, 40

3-1   Insurance Coverage for Immunization by Age Group, 2000, 64
3-2   Public Immunization Funding, Fiscal Years 1999 and 2002, 66
3-3   State Vaccine Purchase Financing Systems, 70
3-4   Insurance Coverage for Immunization and Employer-Based Market Share by Type of Insurance Plan, 71
3-5   Studies of the Impact of Insurance and Cost Sharing on Immunization Rates, 76
3-6   Adults Considered to Be at High Risk for Influenza or Pneumococcal Disease, 88

4-1   Proportion of Publicly Purchased Vaccines Administered in the Private Sector, 93
4-2   Provider Payment for Vaccines and Administration Fees, 98
4-3   Studies on the Impact of Insurance on Referrals, 102

5-1   Domestic Producers of Vaccines for the U.S. Market, 110
5-2   Foreign Producers of Vaccines for the U.S. Market, 112
5-3   Deaths from Selected Diseases Not Yet Preventable by
       Immunization, 119
5-4   Approved Vaccines Withdrawn from the U.S. Market, 123
5-5   Number of Producers of Selected Vaccines for the U.S.
       Market, 2003, 127
5-6   Federal and Private Prices of Vaccines Per Dose, 1983–2002, 130
5-7   Vaccine Supply Status in 2001–2002, 135
5-8   Vaccine Shortages and Their Causes, 136
5-9   Vaccines With and Without Supply Problems, 137

6-1   Summary of Alternative Strategies for Vaccine Purchases, 154

7-1   Legislative Impact of Committee Recommendations, 199
7-2   Proposed Redesign of ACIP Recommendations, 202

FIGURES

1-1   Cumulative vaccine cost trends, 32

2-1   Central role of ACIP in vaccine policy, 58

3-1   Insurance coverage of vaccination, children aged 0–5 (2000), 65
3-2   Insurance coverage of vaccination, adults aged 18–64 (2000), 65

5-1   Federal contract vaccine prices in current dollars, 134

7-1   New vaccine development and subsidy, 188

BOXES

ES-1 Charge to the IOM Committee, 3

1-1   Charge to the IOM Committee, 23

2-1   Vaccine Spillover Effects and Public Good Properties, 42
2-2   Public–Private Collaboration: The Case of DTaP Vaccine, 53

5-1   Vaccine Development and Approval, 115
5-2   Vaccines Expected to Be Developed by 2010, 118

5-3   Vaccine Supply: The Case of DTaP, 125
5-4   Vaccine Purchasing by the Veterans Administration and the
      Department of Defense, 129

6-1   Setting Prices for New Vaccines in Advance, 174

7-1   Calculating the Societal Benefits of Vaccines, 192

FINANCING VACCINES IN THE 21ST CENTURY

Assuring Access and Availability

Executive Summary

ABSTRACT

The public–private partnership that has formed the foundation for purchasing and distributing vaccines in the United States over the past 50 years is showing signs of erosion. The existing national immunization system has performed well in achieving high levels of immunization for children. But difficult new challenges have emerged, including a growing number of recommended vaccines, higher prices associated with new vaccines, persistent disparities in immunization levels, low levels of immunization for adults with chronic illness, the growing burden of immunization on clinicians, recent shortages in the supply of vaccines, and the increasing investment required to license and produce new vaccines.

In addition, the vaccine supply system has undergone radical change. More than 25 companies produced vaccines for the U.S. market in the last 30 years; yet today only 5 companies produce all vaccines recommended for routine use by children and adults. Government purchases now account for more than half of the vaccine market. Government vaccine expenditures are growing rapidly; funding for the Vaccines for Children entitlement program jumped from $500 million to $1 billion between 2000 and 2002 with the addition of new vaccine products to the recommended childhood schedule.

In diagnosing the problems facing the vaccine financing system, the Institute of Medicine's Committee on the Evaluation of Vaccine Purchase Financing in the United States recognized that a strong relationship exists between the system for purchasing and administering vaccines and the stability and growth of the U.S. vaccine supply industry. Although vaccines represent important tools for disease prevention and have significant social value, they frequently generate

1

lower revenues than drugs and other health care services, and provide a less attractive opportunity for private investment in the pharmaceutical industry. To resolve these tensions, the committee recommends strategic reforms that balance public health goals with the need to provide industry a rate of return that is adequate to supply current products and also develop new vaccines. The committee's principal recommendation is the replacement of existing government vaccine purchasing programs with a new vaccine insurance mandate, subsidy, and voucher plan. The mandate would require that all public and private insurance plans include vaccine benefits. The federal government would provide a subsidy to health plans and providers to reimburse their vaccine purchase costs and administration fees. The federal government would also provide vouchers for uninsured children and adults to support recommended immunizations from health care providers of their choice. In formulating this approach, the committee considered several alternative strategies, which are described in the report.

The committee further recommends changes in the composition and decision-making procedures of the Advisory Committee on Immunization Practices, the entity that currently recommends vaccines, to improve the integration of competing objectives within the national immunization system. Finally, the committee recommends the initiation of a deliberative process, an evaluation study, and a research agenda to provide data and indicators that can guide future policy and practice with regard to vaccine financing.

This report presents the results of an evaluation of the financing of vaccine purchases. The purpose of that evaluation was to design a finance strategy that can achieve the right balance in assuring access to the social benefits of vaccines while also encouraging the availability of new and future vaccine products within the health care system. The study was prompted by the publication of an earlier Institute of Medicine (IOM) report, *Calling the Shots* (IOM, 2000a), which examined the financing of immunization infrastructure and recommended a substantial increase ($75 million) in the federal immunization grants program to support infrastructure development. In framing this new study, the Centers for Disease Control and Prevention (CDC) asked the IOM to examine what is known about current vaccine finance arrangements and to identify strategies that could resolve the basic tensions and uncertainties that permeate existing vaccine purchasing systems in the public and private health care sectors. The Committee on the Evaluation of Vaccine Purchase Financing in the United States was formed to conduct this study. The specific charge to the committee, which was based on questions posed by CDC, is shown in Box ES-1.

BOX ES-1
Charge to the IOM Committee

The purpose of the study is to identify financial strategies that are designed to achieve an appropriate balance of roles and responsibilities in the public and private health sectors, integrate federal and state roles in supporting the purchase and administration of recommended vaccines for vulnerable populations, and develop a framework for identifying pricing strategies that can contribute to achieving current and future national immunization goals for children and adults.

The IOM study will develop recommendations to guide federal, state, and congressional decision-making with respect to the purchase of vaccines for the general population, especially underserved groups. The committee will develop a plan that can assure an adequate supply of current vaccines and also provide incentives for the development of new vaccine products. The committee will review factors that influence recent pricing trends in the vaccine industry, identify current health coverage disparities and levels of need that affect access to vaccines in the child and adult populations, and consider the effects of regulatory and licensing procedures on vaccine pricing and vaccine delivery patterns.

BACKGROUND

Immunization represents one of the great triumphs of medical science, one of the most distinctive achievements of the American health care system, and one of the best investments in public health. Vaccines have acquired a special status within the public and private health sectors because they convey significant benefits not only to individuals who are immunized but also to the community at large. Vaccines create a "herd immunity" that protects those who do not receive the vaccine because of medical conditions, those who may be too young to receive the vaccine, those who are not vaccinated because of parental indifference or religious or philosophical objections to vaccination, and those who face financial or other barriers to immunization services. By interrupting the spread of communicable disease, vaccines reduce the number of persons who become infected, diminish the burden of disease, reduce public and private health care expenditures, and improve the quality of life of the general population.

The value of a given vaccine is determined by such factors as protective efficacy, disease incidence, disease outcomes, and costs associated with its use. Moreover, the costs and benefits of individual vaccines vary with the assumptions that guide the assessment of financial and social benefits. Some vaccines produce significant benefits in early childhood; others provide protection during adolescence or adult life. Some vaccines are recommended for universal use; others are recommended only for certain jurisdictions or populations that have specific risk characteristics. Studies have shown that the ratios of vaccination benefits to costs can vary substantially—from 27:1 for diphtheria/pertussis (i.e., $27 worth of benefit for every $1 spent), to 13.5:1 for measles, 4.76:1 for varicella, and 0.68:1–1.1:1 for pneumococcal conjugate.

In general, vaccines are investments that confer significant health and other social benefits. The delivery of recommended vaccines is now a fundamental component of primary health care services for children, and increasingly for adolescents and adults as well. Record high levels of immunization have been achieved for young children; for example, 74 percent of all children now receive the recommended series of vaccines by age 2. Even so, one in four children under age 2 is not up to date on recommended vaccines.

The federal government currently purchases between 52 and 55 percent of the childhood vaccines distributed in the United States, primarily for children who are uninsured or Medicaid-eligible. Nearly 20 doses of vaccines against 11 diseases are required for childhood immunization, at a cost of about $400 at the discounted prices available to the public sector (up to $600 at private-sector prices). This investment strains the ability of both the public and private sectors to immunize a daily birth cohort of more than 11,000 babies. Additional funds are required for the administration of the vaccines, as well as vaccine shipping and storage costs.

In the 10-year period between 1988 and 1997, public-sector expenditures for vaccine purchases doubled from $100 to $200 per child through age 6. The cumulative public-sector cost doubled again in less than 5 years between 1997 and 2001, from $200 to almost $400 per child. The addition to the recommended childhood schedule of the expensive new pneumococcal conjugate vaccine for infants resulted in a doubling of the budget between 2000 and 2002 (from $500 million to over $1 billion in 2000) for the Vaccines for Children (VFC) entitlement—the major government vaccine purchase program for disadvantaged children. Continued cost increases can be expected as a result of the array of new vaccines now in development.

Health officials in both the public and private health care sectors are concerned about the growing fragmentation of effort within the immunization system, as well as the increasing number of recommended vaccines and the high prices of new vaccines. These factors contribute to gaps and uncertainties in health plan benefits for immunization, which can lead in turn to missed opportunities for immunization, greater disparities in immunization rates, and possible outbreaks of vaccine-preventable disease. Moreover, while rates of adult immunization have improved for vaccines that prevent influenza and pneumonia, they are still well below the public health goals established in *Healthy People 2010* (U.S. Department of Health and Human Services, 2000). Adults with chronic health conditions (such as heart and lung disease or diabetes) that place them at high risk for vaccine-preventable disease have particularly low immunization levels.

A public–private partnership has traditionally shared the costs of purchasing and administering vaccines for children, but the private contribution to this partnership may be weakening. While most public and private health plans include vaccine benefits, the scope of those benefits varies widely by type of insurance product and type of vaccine. Federal and state regulations have emerged to require certain types of insurance coverage for some vaccines for children and adults, but the regulatory effort is uneven and difficult to administer. Furthermore, government programs that have been created to provide access to vaccines for children (such as VFC) have not addressed the needs of older adolescents and adults, nor have they created incentives for vaccine administration among health providers.

The uneven nature of health plan vaccine benefits and the limited data on insurance practices with respect to immunization create significant uncertainties in designing national finance strategies for vaccine purchases. The population of underinsured—those who have health care insurance that covers major medical expenses but does not include benefits for vaccines—is a source of increasing concern and uncertainty. Furthermore, some health plans that do include vaccine benefits require out-of-pocket expenses in the form of high deductibles or copayments.

While some states assure access to vaccines for the underinsured, others do not. Some states require immunization coverage in state-regulated insurance plans; others do not. Some states that once had universal purchase policies (thus providing vaccines to all children) are now reducing the scope of their benefits.

Recent vaccine shortages that were unprecedented in their scope and severity, as well as diminishing numbers of vaccine suppliers for the U.S. market, are early warning signs of other problems that require systemic remedies to assure a healthy and reliable vaccine supply system. While temporary production problems appear to have eased, the potential for disruption remains. The problem of vaccine shortages has raised concerns about the relationships among the size of the government vaccine market, low vaccine prices, and the scale of investment in the production of current vaccines and the development of new vaccine products. The ability of the government to negotiate low prices for recommended vaccines is important to public health agencies and others that are trying to stretch tight budgets to cover both traditional vaccines and a growing array of new and higher-priced vaccine products. On the other hand, adequate financial incentives are necessary to sustain private investment in the vaccine production and licensing processes if the vaccine industry is to remain competitive and have the capacity to innovate within a global vaccine market.

Incremental reforms have been offered to solve discrete aspects of the problems associated with access to and the supply of current vaccines. For example, the proposed fiscal year 2004 federal budget includes proposals to increase the scope of the safety net, lift vaccine price caps, and expand the size of vaccine stockpiles. These reforms may provide temporary relief from acute problems, but the nation still lacks a comprehensive finance strategy that can adapt to expected increases in both the number and prices of vaccines, continue to assure access for disadvantaged populations, and also sustain incentives for private investment in the production and licensing of current and future vaccine products.

CONCLUSIONS

Routine immunization for recommended vaccines, especially for children, is achieved through a partnership between public health clinics and private clinicians. In formulating the following conclusions, the committee focused on aspects of the immunization system that represent important sources of stress and tension associated with current vaccine purchase practices. Other aspects of the immunization system (such as concerns about the quality of the public health infrastructure, vaccine safety issues, military vaccines, and the role of vaccines in dealing with bioterrorism) are addressed in other IOM reports (IOM, 2000a,b; 2002a,b,c; 2003).

Conclusion 1: Current public and private financing strategies for immunization have had substantial success, especially in improving immunization rates for young children. However, significant disparities remain in assuring access to recommended vaccines across geographic and demographic populations.

Despite improvements, current childhood immunization levels (about 74 percent of all 2-year-old children) have not achieved the national health goal of 80 percent immunization. One in four young children is not up to date in receiving recommended immunizations.

Substantial variation (almost 20 percent) in immunization rates currently exists within and across states. Some large urban centers, in particular, have low immunization rates for children aged 19 to 36 months.

The specific causes of these disparities are not well understood, but low levels of immunization are commonly associated with areas characterized by a concentration of poverty and populations that frequently move in and out of safety net programs.

In addition, the disparities between children and adults in the burden of vaccine–preventable disease are troubling. Although the reported use of pneumococcal and influenza vaccines among adults aged 65 and older more than doubled in the period 1988–1995, morbidity and mortality for both diseases remain significant in this population. Immunization rates for high-risk adults (aged 18–64) with chronic disease are especially poor: in 1999, 31.9 percent received an annual influenza vaccination, while only 17.1 percent had ever received a pneumococcal vaccination. The difficulties associated with risk-based strategies (i.e., based on health conditions) for adults have caused many providers within the health profession to shift to an age-based strategy to encourage vaccination of adults.

Conclusion 2: Substantial increases can be expected to occur in public and private health expenditures as new vaccine products become available. While these cost increases will be offset by the health and other social benefits associated with these advances in vaccine development, the growing costs of vaccines will be increasingly burdensome to all health sectors. Alternatives to current vaccine pricing and purchasing programs are required to sustain stable investment in the development of new vaccine products and attain their social benefits for all.

Although the costs associated with purchasing and delivering vaccines have historically been small, new vaccines will be priced at higher levels reflecting the scale of investment necessary to bring new products through the licensing and production processes. The addition of new vaccines to the recommended schedule and the higher costs associated with newer vaccine products have placed tremendous stress on safety net programs that are already straining to achieve public health goals. Higher vaccine prices can be expected to exacerbate such problems as uneven distribution patterns, delays in the vaccine price negotiation processes for federal and state contracts, and continued fragmentation in the scope of vaccine benefits included in public and private health plans. An increased burden on public health clinics also occurs when private health plans reduce reimbursements for recommended vaccines in the face of higher costs. This burden places substantial stress on public health budgets and interferes with the ability to provide vaccines to traditional safety net populations, as well as those who lack vaccine benefits within their health plans.

It should be noted that vaccines provide a net long-term savings in health care costs. Over time, vaccines should lead to a diminution in what would otherwise be spent on health care. But certain sectors (such as state and federal health agencies) will bear substantial short-term costs of acquiring and delivering vaccines.

Increases in the budgets of government vaccine programs should be seen as acceptable, indeed desirable, insofar as new vaccines can offer substantial public health benefits. What is missing in the array of current vaccine purchasing programs is a clear and deliberate strategy that the government can use to stabilize and assure adequate rates of return on future private investments in vaccine development. While the true costs of innovation remain unknown, government pricing systems and bulk purchases alone appear to provide insufficient incentives, according to industry sources, given the higher production costs and uncertainties associated with vaccine development and the tendency to push down prices in the public sector.

Conclusion 3: Many young children, adolescents, and high-risk adults have no or limited insurance for recommended vaccines. Gaps and fragmentation in insurance benefits create barriers for both vulnerable populations and clinicians that can contribute to lower immunization rates.

As noted above, many individuals are underinsured—their health insurance benefits do not include coverage for immunization. Estimates of underinsurance among children vary from 5 to 14 percent. Others have insurance policies that require individuals to share the costs of vaccines in the form of high deductibles and copayments. Still others, such as Medicare beneficiaries, are covered for certain vaccines but not others. Persons who face such financial barriers are less likely to receive routine immunizations in their medical homes and may fail to receive certain immunizations at all.

Although most large public and private health plans include vaccine benefits, signs of slippage are occurring within the scope of vaccine benefits offered by small businesses and other large subscribers, such as public employee health plans. The omission of or limitations on vaccine benefits in health plans, coupled with increasing deductibles and copayments, create gaps that existing safety net programs cannot easily fill. The result is increasing fragmentation and administrative barriers that interfere with the timely delivery of vaccines within routine health care services.

The multifaceted eligibility determinations associated with the current fragmented system of public and private vaccine benefits impose substantial burdens on clinicians. Clinicians must determine whether the costs of purchasing and administering recommended vaccines are reimbursable under the terms of a wide variety of insurance plans and entitlements, including VFC, the State Children's Health Insurance Program (SCHIP), CDC's Section 317 program, Medicare, and multiple private health insurance plans. These administrative barriers can result in missed opportunities for immunization and frequent referrals of underinsured patients to public health clinics for routine vaccines, which in turn contribute to shortfalls in immunization rates.

Conclusion 4: Current government strategies for purchasing and assuring access to recommended vaccines have not addressed the relationships between the financing of vaccine purchases and the stability of the U.S. vaccine supply. Financial incentives are necessary to protect the existing supply of vaccine products, as well as to encourage the development of new vaccine products.

Significant tensions exist in the vaccine supply system between the need to control public and private expenditures on vaccines and the need to encourage investment in the production and development of current and future vaccines. While a series of stopgap proposals and measures has emerged in recent years to address recurring tensions, no coordinated strategy exists to balance the goals of assuring access to vaccines and sustaining the supply of vaccine products. The result is an unstable market that reduces incentives for future vaccine development and threatens to exacerbate current structural problems within the industry.

Conclusion 5: The vaccine recommendation process does not adequately incorporate consideration of a vaccine's price and societal benefits.

The recommendations of the Advisory Committee on Immunization Practices (ACIP) and its counterpart groups within the American Academy of Pediatrics and the American Academy of Family Practitioners have significant implications for public and private expenditures. For example, ACIP recommendations directly affect vaccine prices and supply, such as the addition of vaccine products to the recommended vaccine schedule, the inclusion of vaccines in the VFC entitlement program, the standard of care for the Medicaid vaccine schedule, and the universal purchase guidelines for many states. Yet the ACIP decision-making process requires the formulation of recommendations before the government purchase price has been negotiated. In addition, ACIP has no mechanism for distinguishing vaccines with strong spillover effects, such as those that prevent highly contagious diseases, from vaccines that do not, such as tetanus and certain therapeutic vaccines that are in development. The lack of a capacity to address these variables is a serious impediment to a coherent finance strategy for vaccine purchases in the national immunization system.

ALTERNATIVE STRATEGIES

In framing its recommendations, the committee focused its analysis on seven alternative approaches, which included market-oriented, government intervention, and incremental strategies. Each approach was considered in terms of its impact on both access to vaccines and incentives for the production and development of vaccines in the private sector. In addition, the committee sought to design a strategy that would maintain a reasonable budget for vaccine purchases for children and adults in the public and private health sectors. The following alternative approaches were considered:

1. Maintain the current system.
2. Expand the VFC program to include additional eligibility categories.
3. Provide universal coverage through federal purchase and supply of all recommended vaccines.
4. Provide a federal block grant to the states for vaccine purchase.
5. Use public vouchers to purchase recommended vaccines for disadvantaged populations.
6. Create an insurance mandate that would require public and private health plans to cover all recommended vaccines.
7. Combine features of the insurance mandate and voucher alternatives into a new funded mandate system.

Each of these alternatives has certain advantages in assuring access to recommended vaccines. However, the committee concluded that alternative 7 has the greatest potential to assure access while also offering incentives for the development and production of vaccines. Incremental reforms that perpetuate the current fragmentation may help resolve one crisis or strengthen an isolated component of a dynamic and interactive system, but such piecemeal approaches do not foster a coherent strategy that can align national health policy goals with the desired outcomes. It was the consensus of the committee that to maintain the current system without fundamental reforms would ultimately result in deterioration of the immunization system and weaken incentives for future vaccine research and production. Requiring insurance coverage for immunization, for example, could lead to higher premiums and cost-sharing practices that might reduce access to vaccines or shift larger numbers of individuals to government programs. A universal purchase proposal would also be problematic if governmental expansion within the vaccine market led to lower prices and discouraged private investment in new vaccine products. Such issues point to the need for close attention to the ways in which escalating costs shift the immunization burden between the public and private health sectors and between individuals and health plans.

RECOMMENDATIONS

Ultimately, the committee determined that the best strategy would be to formulate a comprehensive plan that can address multiple goals. This plan would encompass a mandated insurance benefit strategy that includes a subsidy for insurers; a decentralized, private market for vaccines; and a voucher program for the uninsured. The committee formulated its strategy in three recommendations.

Recommendation 1: The committee recommends the implementation of a new insurance mandate, combined with a government subsidy and voucher plan, for vaccines recommended by the Advisory Committee on Immunization Practices (ACIP).

The proposed plan, referred to as the *vaccine payment system,* consists of five core components that should be considered an integrated strategy for achieving the key objectives of access to and availability of vaccines:

• Federal legislation would be required to establish a vaccination coverage mandate for all public and private health plans. This mandate would apply to both state-regulated insurance plans and self-funded employer plans (which are exempt from state regulation under the Employee Retirement Income Security Act [ERISA]), as well as Medicare, Medicaid, SCHIP, and government health plans for military personnel and civilian employees. The mandate would provide coverage for all insured children; adults aged 65 and older; and certain designated populations, such as adults aged 18–64 who have certain health disorders that place them at higher risk for vaccine-preventable disease.
• The federal government would create a new federal subsidy to reimburse public and private health plans and providers for mandated vaccine costs and associated vaccine administration fees.
• The federal government would also create a voucher system for vaccines and vaccine administration fees for designated uninsured populations.
• The insurance mandate, subsidy, and voucher would apply principally to vaccines that have substantial spillover effects as a result of their

ability to prevent highly contagious diseases. Vaccines without substantial spillover effects, such as therapeutic vaccines, would be considered for inclusion only in cases of exceptional societal benefit.

• The amount of the subsidy and voucher would be determined both for vaccines currently on the immunization schedule and for vaccines that are not yet available. The subsidy for new vaccines would be based on an estimate of their societal benefit. The subsidy for vaccines already in use would be based on a formula that would take into account both current market prices and the vaccines' calculated societal benefit. The mandate would not apply to vaccines priced above the subsidy amount.

Major Features. A government-funded insurance mandate for immunization represents a reformulation of a universal vaccine purchase program and would assure that clinically appropriate immunization services would become a basic and required feature of all public and private health insurance plans. This strategy changes the role of government from one of buying vaccines to one of assuring immunization by mandating insurance coverage for recommended vaccines, as well as providing a fixed subsidy adequate to reimburse both vaccine purchase costs and administration fees for public and private insurers and clinicians. As a universal program, the government vaccine subsidy is extended to all persons within the designated populations. As a payment reimbursement program, it sustains the role of government in subsidizing the cost of immunization and enhances incentives for investment in vaccine products, but it reduces the impact of government purchases on the vaccine market relative to other approaches (such as a universal purchase policy).

The prospect of a guaranteed public subsidy for selected vaccines would provide economic incentives that would encourage manufacturers to invest in the clinical trial, licensing, and production processes necessary to move a vaccine product from the early stage of discovery to its use in routine medical care. Reducing the financial uncertainties associated with these processes would stimulate the market and encourage the development of new and effective vaccine products.

At the same time, the federal subsidy for vaccines would not provide a blank check for a new vaccine product. The process of establishing a predetermined subsidy for vaccines not yet licensed would offer incentives for reliable and innovative vaccine product development while also encouraging efficiency and competition in the production process. Specific advantages and limitations of the recommended strategy are discussed below.

Advantages. The proposed vaccine payment plan has several clear advantages. The plan would:

• Improve incentives for the development of new vaccines by providing manufacturers with assurance of adequate pricing and returns for those vaccines that confer substantial public benefit.

• Increase immunization rates by eliminating or reducing barriers to access associated with vaccine costs or health insurance benefits.

• Create a more pluralistic market for vaccines that would encourage health care providers and health plans to purchase vaccines best suited to the needs of their patients and subscribers.

• Build upon the strengths of the current arrangements of public and private health plans and avoid the creation of separate or parallel programs.

• Eliminate the economic distortions and administrative barriers associated with the direct federal purchase of vaccines.

• Reduce the role of government in purchasing vaccines and avoid delays now associated with eligibility standards, protracted contract negotiations, price caps, discretionary funding cycles, and discount arrangements.

• Reduce the potential for passing higher vaccine costs on to individuals.

• Support the administration of vaccines within individuals' medical homes and strengthen the bond between immunization and other primary health care services.

• Support the rapid uptake of new recommended vaccines and reduce the disparities and fragmentation now associated with the time delays involved in negotiating contracts and budgets for federal vaccine purchases.

• Sustain the partnership among governments (federal, state, and local), health plans, health care providers, and vaccine companies in achieving the societal benefits of disease prevention.

• Maintain a market-oriented pricing approach.

Disadvantages. Four disadvantages are associated with the proposed vaccine payment system:

• Federal expenditures for vaccines would increase, primarily because of expanded public coverage for vaccines as a result of the insurance mandate.

• The replacement of a government purchase price with a federal subsidy could result in higher prices for some vaccine products.

• Setting a subsidy for vaccines not yet licensed based on a calculation of societal benefit, without reference to market forces, would require the development of a consistent methodology to resolve numerous technical difficulties. Controversies could arise in assigning monetary values to life-years and quality of life as part of the societal benefit calculations. Substantial legislative and regulatory guidance, in addition to expert guidance and public debate, could be required to resolve these controversies.

• Implementation of the vaccine payment plan would require substantial amendments to the laws and regulations governing various public and private health plans (e.g., ERISA, the Public Health Act, Medicare, Medicaid, and SCHIP). A comprehensive legislative strategy would be necessary to reduce the risk of an incremental and uneven approach.

> **Recommendation 2: The Secretary of the Department of Health and Human Services should propose changes in the procedures and membership of ACIP so that its recommendations can associate vaccine coverage decisions with societal benefits and costs, including consideration of the impact of the price of a vaccine on recommendations for its use.**

The Secretary of DHHS should develop rules that address both the ACIP membership and decision-making process. These rules would modify current practices through administrative action or legislation, where necessary.

ACIP Membership. Voting membership in ACIP should be expanded to include expertise in health insurance benefit design, public and private health care delivery systems, consumer issues (including concerns regarding vulnerable populations, such as disabled persons, racial and ethnic minorities, and rural populations), health economics and finance, cost–benefit assessment, and vaccine manufacturing. The representation of these perspectives is essential to inform ACIP decision making with respect to the impact of vaccine price and coverage on population groups, providers, payors, and other key stakeholders. At the same time, it is important to maintain the independence and balance that have traditionally guided ACIP recommendation procedures through a rigorous and transparent conflict and bias screening process for voting members. Current employees or agents of firms within the insurance and vaccine manufacturing industries should not participate as voting members, although access to their expertise is necessary to inform committee deliberations.

Immunization Schedule Determinations. ACIP should continue its present practice of recommending current and new vaccines for universal or selected populations within the immunization schedule. These determinations should be based on a vaccine's efficacy, safety, cost-effectiveness (reflecting current price information), feasibility, supply, and other considerations.

Mandate and Subsidy Determinations. In addition, ACIP should determine whether a vaccine has sufficient spillover effects to warrant its inclusion in the new insurance mandate and subsidy category. The mandate determination for new vaccines would require a judgment about the extent to which a vaccine offers societal benefits beyond its value to the vaccinated individual. An important criterion in determining societal benefits should be the extent to which immunization conveys herd immunity. The mandate should apply principally to vaccines with substantial spillover effects. However, other vaccines, such as therapeutic vaccines, would be considered for inclusion in cases of exceptional social benefit, such as when disparities in immunization rates between insured and uninsured persons persist for a substantial time after licensure of a vaccine.

Once a vaccine had been selected for inclusion under the insurance mandate as discussed in recommendation 1, ACIP would calculate the monetary value of the federal subsidy for reimbursement to public and private insurers. This calculation would be based on a methodology that would assign values to such factors as reduced health expenditures, enhanced quality of life, and increased labor productivity.

The mandate and subsidy process would apply to both current and future vaccines. Future vaccines should receive primary consideration to stimulate the development of new vaccine products. Current ACIP-recommended vaccine components, such as tetanus, could be "grandfathered" into the mandate and subsidy category to avoid confusion and disruptions to the current vaccine schedule and immunization system.

Staff support for these new functions and the redesigned ACIP would require expansion of the supporting responsibilities of the National Vaccine Program Office and the National Immunization Program within CDC.

Recommendation 3: As part of the implementation of recommendations 1 and 2, the National Vaccine Program Office should convene a series of stakeholder deliberations on the administrative, technical, and legislative issues associated with a shift from vaccine purchase to a vaccine mandate, subsidy, and voucher finance strategy. In addition, the Centers for Disease Control and Prevention (CDC) should sponsor a postimplementation evaluation study (in 5 years, for example). CDC should also initiate a research program aimed at improving the measurement of the societal value of vaccines, addressing methodological challenges, and providing a basis for comparing the impact of different measurement approaches in achieving national immunization goals.

Recommendations 1 and 2 represent a significant departure from current law and practice. A change of this magnitude is warranted to address the fundamental and systemic problems that confront the national immunization system. Piecemeal changes are unlikely to solve these problems. Incremental reforms also are incapable of achieving an appropriate balance between access and availability in vaccine financing.

In formulating its recommendations, the committee has sketched the broad outlines of long-term strategic reforms. These recommendations do not address all aspects of the shift from the existing vaccine purchase programs to a mandate, subsidy, and voucher plan, nor do they incorporate the comprehensive legislative agenda that would be necessary to achieve these reforms. A major national debate and examination of the committee's proposals among diverse stakeholders is necessary prior to full implementation of these recommendations.

The committee therefore urges the National Vaccine Program Office to organize a series of public meetings with key experts and interest groups, including health plans, providers, vaccine industry representatives, public health officials, and others, to address how the proposed arrangements might be implemented through a staged roll-out informed by further data and analysis. These discussions should address the following topics:

- *What populations should be included in the vaccine payment plan?* The federal vaccine payment plan is envisioned primarily as a means of addressing the immunization needs of young children, older adults, and high-risk adults between the ages of 18 and 64. The inclusion of other populations—such as all adolescents (under age 21) and all adults, regardless of their health condition—should be considered as well. The initial purpose of the expanded coverage is to target public finance toward those who are currently underserved. A second goal, which supports the proposal for universal coverage of all children and adults, is to reduce the current fragmentation in vaccine coverage that leads to gaps and administrative burdens in determining eligibility, and to foster efficiency in providing access to vaccines that are delivered primarily in private health care settings. The means by which vaccines would be delivered to and reimbursed for different groups might differ by age, employment circumstances, and access to health care services.

- *How would the insurance mandate and subsidy system operate?* The insurance mandate would apply to all public and private insurers, including ERISA and ERISA-exempt plans, Medicaid, SCHIP, Medicare, and other public insurance (such as CHAMPUS) and public health programs (such as that of the Indian Health Service). The mandate could extend to all insured persons within these health plans or only to selected populations, such as young children, older adults, and high-risk groups. The voucher system would provide access to vaccines for all uninsured people in these categories. For some programs, current program dollars for vaccine purchases and vaccine administration would be replaced by the vaccine payment system dollars. For example, vaccines administered through Medicaid and SCHIP would no longer be funded through those programs' federal–state matching funds but through the new centralized vaccine system. Medicare would also be included in the mandate; but for purposes of administrative efficiency, Medicare vaccination would be paid for by that program's own funds.

• *How should societal value be calculated?* This report defines the societal value of a vaccine as its total benefits, including both the private benefits to the person receiving it and the benefits to others. Using this approach, a monetary value is assigned to all benefits associated with a new vaccine that can be determined and measured (for example, future medical costs that are averted, as well as additional life-years and enhanced quality of life). The sum of these values represents the vaccine's societal benefit. As noted above in the discussion of disadvantages, this calculation involves certain technical challenges. Developing a consistent methodology and making assumptions explicit for all vaccines would be of value in the decision-making process not only for vaccines but in other spheres of health care as well. Changes in the benefit calculation should be expected as knowledge of a vaccine's immunogenicity and the impact of other therapeutic effects on disease outcomes improves over time.

• *How would the calculated societal benefit be used to determine the subsidy amount?* The creation of a predetermined subsidy for future vaccines is intended to be an incentive to stimulate private-sector investment in vaccine development. Determining the amount of the subsidy would require a calculation of the societal benefit of each future vaccine, but the value of the subsidy would not necessarily equal the full value of the societal benefit. While the subsidy should not exceed the societal value of the vaccine product, it should also not be so low that it fails to serve as an adequate incentive for research and development. Different approaches might be considered, such as adopting a fixed standard (for example, 90 percent of the societal value) or limiting the range of new vaccine prices to some multiple of current prices.

• *How would the subsidy for current vaccines be determined?* The calculation of a subsidy for current vaccines would require consideration of both the societal value of the vaccine product and recent market prices. Some vaccines might receive a subsidy significantly higher than current prices if judged to be undervalued in terms of their societal benefit. Adjustments to the value of the subsidy might also be warranted to account for inflation, as well as changes in the costs of production or regulatory compliance.

• *Who would administer the subsidy and voucher system?* The vaccine payment system is designed to serve multiple objectives: to address the vaccine needs of vulnerable populations, to assure a reliable supply of current and future vaccines by diversifying the vaccine purchasing market, and to relieve clinicians of the administrative burden of determining individual eligibility for vaccines. Ideally, one federal agency within DHHS would be responsible for administering the subsidy and voucher system, as well as overseeing compliance with the insurance mandate for vaccine coverage. Certain responsibilities might be delegated to state agencies (in such areas as insurance regulation and administration of the voucher plan), but a central coordinating strategy would be required to assure consistent eligibility criteria and practices throughout the states.

• *How would the proposed mandate treat deductibles and copayments?* While many states have mandated first-dollar coverage for vaccines, immunization costs might apply toward the general deductible that is customary practice for health plans. While many current vaccines are inexpensive, significant price increases can be expected in the future. Cost sharing could encourage consumers to shop for efficient providers and help control inflationary pressures; however, it could adversely affect immunization rates should financial factors become burdensome for the consumer. The extent to which cost sharing should be included in the vaccine payment plan would require further consideration in the implementation process.

Evaluation Plan. The magnitude and uncertainties of the changes associated with the recommended vaccine payment system are significant. The committee recommends that an evaluation study be included as part of the implementation plan to address certain key issues. Specifically, this study should include an analysis of the impact of the mandate and subsidy in two distinct areas: access to vaccines and the availability of the vaccine supply.

In the first area, data should be gathered on how the payment system affects the delivery of vaccines to selected population groups (insured, uninsured, and underinsured), age cohorts (young children and high-risk adults), and geographic settings (rural and urban), possibly through demonstration studies aimed at identifying key challenges involved in the implementation process in selected states. The costs of implementation, outreach, education, reimbursement, and oversight should be measured to determine how to gain greater efficiencies in administering the program.

In the second area, the impact of the diversified market and predetermined subsidy plan should be examined in light of their relationship to private investments in the production and licensing of new vaccine products. The evaluation study should consider the assumptions that guide the calculations of social benefit, as well as other data that influence the level of vaccine subsidy and voucher payments.

The positive and negative effects of replacing current safety net programs with the proposed government-funded mandate are unknown and could be significant. The VFC entitlement and Section 317 vaccine purchase program have been productive tools in improving immunization levels within the public sector. These programs have a history of strong bipartisan support and effective delivery of vaccines for disadvantaged populations, especially during difficult fiscal times; but they are also associated with disruptions in supply and a decrease in the number of vaccine manufacturers. Similarly, state-supported vaccine purchase programs are often the foundation of safety net immunization efforts in certain jurisdictions. Strategies need to be developed to assure that the payment plan advocated here will at least sustain and ideally improve current immunization rates among disadvantaged populations.

Research Agenda. Addressing many of the issues examined in this report will require further understanding of the ways in which basic market forces interact with access to and the delivery of vaccines to children, adolescents, and adults. Limited data are available to support rigorous examination of such empirical questions as the relationship of insurance benefits to immunization status. More funding is needed to support research studies that can monitor the extent to which pricing, supply, mandates, and other health policy and health finance factors influence the performance and outcomes of immunization efforts. Suggested topics for an initial set of research studies include the following:

- The numbers and characteristics of children and adults having public or private insurance benefits that include immunization and the types of restrictions on their immunization benefits.
- The impact of insurance status (both public and private) and cost-sharing arrangements on the timing and setting of vaccine administration and immunization status.
- The impact of alternative vaccine payment arrangements on clinician behavior and referral rates for immunization.
- The effect of full or partial subsidies on the supply and delivery of childhood and adult vaccines.
- The relationship between vaccine prices and supplier investments in research and development.
- The relationship between U.S. and global vaccine production, supply, regulation, and prices.

FINAL OBSERVATIONS

The findings, alternative strategies, and recommendations set forth in this report provide a blueprint to guide the nation's public and private health sectors in adapting to foreseeable changes in vaccine development in the decades ahead. The public and private partnership that supports the immunization of children and adults in the United States requires vigilance and flexibility in assuring that the social benefits of vaccines will continue to be available to all, regardless of ability to pay or health care setting. Assuring access and sustaining incentives that contribute to the availability of safe and effective vaccines are the twin goals that must guide vaccine finance strategies in the 21st century.

1

Introduction

This report presents the results of an evaluation of the financing of vaccine purchases. The purpose of that evaluation was to design a finance strategy that can achieve the right balance in assuring access to the social benefits of vaccines while also encouraging the availability of new and future vaccine products within the health care system. The study was prompted by the publication of an earlier Institute of Medicine (IOM) report, *Calling the Shots* (Institute of Medicine [IOM], 2000a), which examined the financing of immunization infrastructure and recommended a substantial increase ($75 million) in the federal immunization grants program to support infrastructure development. In framing this new study, the Centers for Disease Control and Prevention (CDC) asked the IOM to examine what is known about current vaccine finance arrangements and to identify strategies that could resolve the basic tensions and uncertainties that permeate existing vaccine purchasing systems in the public and private health care sectors. The Committee on the Evaluation of Vaccine Purchase Financing in the United States was formed to conduct this study.

CDC formulated the following questions as the basic framework for this study:

(1) What are the roles and responsibilities of public (federal, state, and local) and private (health plans, health insurers, and purchasers) agencies and health care providers in financing the purchase of vaccines to achieve national immunization objectives for all children, adolescents, and adults in the U.S.?

(a) Who is responsible for payment of costs for all vaccines for children, adolescents, and adults licensed by the Food and Drug Administration (FDA) and recommended by the Advisory Committee on Immunization Practices (ACIP)?

(b)   How can public and private prices of a new vaccine be determined in a rapid and fair manner to balance the need for continued investment in vaccine research with the financial constraints of the health care system in the United States?

(2)   In working toward an appropriate balance of roles and responsibilities, which finance strategies best achieve national goals and best fit the service delivery mechanisms for various vaccines and/or population groups?

(a)   What are the public health and cost implications of these alternatives?

(b)   How can these strategies be implemented given limited resources for preventive health interventions?

(3)   What are the current levels of need for recommended vaccines in the child, adolescent, and adult populations for those persons who do not have health plan benefits that include immunizations or who have large co-payments and/or deductibles?

(a)   What changes in the level of need are anticipated in the future?

(4)   Which approaches could reduce the time lag and disparities that occur between new vaccine recommendations and the availability of public and private financing to implement the recommendation?

(5)   Will vaccine products under consideration for licensing have a significant effect on future vaccine purchase strategies in public and private health plans?

(a)   Why have vaccine prices increased in the past decade?

(b)   What lessons have been learned in other fields with finance systems that purchase medical devices or supplies from single manufacturers?

These broad study questions were translated into the charge for the IOM committee, shown in Box 1-1.

BACKGROUND

Vaccines are a fundamental component of primary health care services, especially for children. Building on basic research discoveries, a growing number of vaccine products are now available that provide protection against once-common infectious diseases across the lifespan. The widespread use of available vaccines in the United States has led to significant declines in the mortality and morbidity rates associated with such

BOX 1-1
Charge to the IOM Committee

The purpose of the study is to identify financial strategies that are designed to achieve an appropriate balance of roles and responsibilities in the public and private health sectors, integrate federal and state roles in supporting the purchase and administration of recommended vaccines for vulnerable populations, and develop a framework for identifying pricing strategies that can contribute to achieving current and future national immunization goals for children and adults.

The IOM study will develop recommendations to guide federal, state, and congressional decision-making with respect to the purchase of vaccines for the general population, especially underserved groups. The committee will develop a plan that can assure an adequate supply of current vaccines and also provide incentives for the development of new vaccine products. The committee will review factors that influence recent pricing trends in the vaccine industry, identify current health coverage disparities and levels of need that affect access to vaccines in the child and adult populations, and consider the effects of regulatory and licensing procedures on vaccine pricing and vaccine delivery patterns.

illnesses as polio, measles, mumps, rubella, pertussis, diphtheria, smallpox, tetanus, influenza, and pneumonia (see Table 1-1). Measurements of immunization status are frequently used as benchmarks in determining the health status of an individual child, as well as in assessing the health status of populations of children and adults (see Appendix A for the childhood and adult immunization schedules for 2002–2003).

Current reports (Centers for Disease Control and Prevention [CDC], 2002a) indicate that 73.7 percent of all U.S. children (aged 19 to 35 months) have received the full schedule of vaccines recommended for their age group (4:3:1:3:3 series).[1] This rate has remained relatively stable over the past 3 years. A higher percentage of children (close to or even more than 90 percent) has received a significant portion of the recommended vac-

---

[1]The 4:3:1:3:3 series, which constituted the universal recommended schedule in 2001, comprises 4 doses of diphtheria–tetanus–acellular pertussis vaccine, 3 doses of poliovirus vaccine, 1 dose of measles-containing vaccine, 3 doses of hepatitis B vaccine, and 3 doses of *haemophilus influenzae* type b vaccine. Varicella and pneumococcal conjugate vaccines are measured separately.

TABLE 1-1 Change in Annual Morbidity from Vaccine-Preventable Diseases: Prevaccine Baseline and 2002

Disease	Prevaccine Baseline Date	Average Annual Baseline Cases	2002 Cases[a]	% Decrease
Diphtheria	1920–1922	175,885	1	100.0
Haemophilus influenzae, type b and unknown[a]	1985	20,000	167	99.2
Measles	1958–1962	503,282	37	100.0
Mumps	1968	152,209	238	99.8
Pertussis	1922–1925	147,271	8,296	94.4
Invasive pneumococcal[b]	1998–1999	13,330	2,700	80
Poliomyelitis	1951–1954	16,316	0	100.0
Rubella	1966–1968	47,745	14	100.0
Congenital Rubella Syndrome	1998	823	3	99.6
Tetanus	1922–1926	1,314	22	98.3

[a]Children <5 years old.
[b]Children <2 years old; preliminary data from CDC's Active Bacterial Core Surveillance/ Emerging Infections Program Network.
NOTE: Preliminary 2002 (52-week frozen) data.
SOURCES: IOM, 2000a; CDC, 2003a.

cines by 24 months of age[2] (CDC, 2003b), and virtually all children (about 95 percent) are adequately immunized by the time they enter school. Those who are not immunized by school age are frequently from families that have requested an exemption from immunization requirements for medical, religious, or philosophical reasons.

These high rates of immunization among young children are impressive. By these measures, the United States has developed a successful immunization system for children that provides significant protection against vaccine-preventable disease. Yet several fundamental concerns remain.

First, the public health goal of 80 percent immunization of 2-year-old children with recommended vaccines has never been achieved. While outbreaks of vaccine-preventable disease have decreased significantly, full immunization of the young, and especially vulnerable child populations, with all

---

[2]The reported percentages are as follows: 94 percent receive 3 of the 4 recommended diphtheria-pertussis-tetanus (DPT) vaccines; 88 percent receive 3 polio vaccines; 90 percent receive 1 measles-mumps-rubella (MMR) vaccine; 93 percent receive 3 Haemophilus influenzae type b (HIB) vaccines; and 89 percent receive 3 of the newer hepatitis B vaccines.

recommended vaccines remains elusive. One of every four 2-year-old children in the United States is not adequately immunized. Public health officials have established clear standards to strengthen immunization efforts at the national, state, and local levels. These standards, which are set forth in the report *Healthy People 2010* (U.S. Department of Health and Human Services, 2000), establish a national goal of 80 percent immunization with recommended vaccines for all 2-year-old children.

Second, broad disparities remain in state and local immunization rates for young children. There is substantial variation in immunization rates among states. According to data collected by the 2001 National Immunization Survey (NIS), Rhode Island had the highest level of immunization for children aged 19–35 months (81.7 percent for the 4:3:1:3:3 series). New Mexico ranked lowest for the same series (63.2 percent), a difference of more than 18 percentage points (CDC, 2002a).

Significant variations also exist among urban areas and between urban and state-level rates. The highest estimated rate of immunization of young children (aged 19–35 months, 4:3:1:3:3 series) in the 2001 NIS data was 79.5 percent in Jefferson County, Alabama, compared with a low rate of 57.7 percent in Detroit, Michigan—a difference of 21.8 percentage points (CDC, 2002a). Similar disparities were revealed within states as well. Michigan, for example, had a state-level immunization rate of 71.7 percent, 14 percentage points higher than the rate for the city of Detroit. Similarly, the state-level rate for New Jersey was 73.8 percent, as compared with a rate of 58.8 percent for Newark—a difference of 15 percentage points.

While cities such as Boston and San Diego enjoy high immunization rates as compared with the national average of 73.7 percent for all U.S. children aged 19 to 35 months, other cities are struggling. In addition to Newark and Detroit, cities that reported low levels of immunization for young children included Washington, D.C. (68.9 percent), Baltimore (65.3 percent), Philadelphia (64.9 percent), Houston (63.0 percent), and Dallas (63.1 percent) (CDC, 2002a).

Third, a significant burden of vaccine-preventable disease remains within the adult population. Adults experience the highest levels of mortality and morbidity from vaccine-preventable diseases. Influenza and pneumonia are the seventh leading cause of death in the United States, responsible for more than 65,000 deaths annually—most among older adults (CDC, 2002b).[3] In contrast, about 300 deaths occur each year as a result of all

---

[3]Note, however, that the majority of these deaths are among those aged 65 and above. Some percentage of these deaths are likely due to family decisions not to immunize because of extreme age or comorbidities.

vaccine-preventable diseases among children. In addition, 48,000 pneumonia and influenza hospitalizations occur annually among adults over age 65 (CDC, 2001a). The monetary burden of adult vaccine-preventable diseases is estimated to be greater than $10 billion per year (CDC, 2002c). The annual immunization rates for noninstitutionalized adults age 65 and older are 66 percent for influenza vaccine and 50 percent for pneumococcal vaccines (CDC, 2002d). The missed opportunities for immunization represented by these figures carry a high and avoidable cost for individuals and society as a whole, especially among older adults.

Finally, working-age adults with chronic illnesses have persistently low levels of immunization that place them at risk. Immunization rates for high-risk adults who suffer from chronic disease (e.g., heart or lung disease or diabetes) are especially low. A national health objective for 2010 is to increase influenza and pneumococcal vaccination rates to at least 60 percent among persons at high risk for complications from these diseases.[4] The Advisory Committee on Immunization Practices (ACIP) has recommended, for example, that all persons with diabetes be vaccinated. Yet recent data indicate that only 40 percent of persons with diabetes had received an influenza vaccination within the previous year, and only 21 percent had ever received a pneumococcal vaccination (CDC, 1999a). Validated immunization estimates for other recommended adult vaccines (e.g., hepatitis A, hepatitis B, tetanus, and varicella) are severely limited or nonexistent (IOM, 2000a). In addition to generally low immunization rates among adults, significant racial and ethnic disparities persist in adult immunization levels (CDC, 2002d).

CONCEPTUAL FRAMEWORK FOR THE STUDY

Investments in research and development throughout the 20th century have generated a growing array of vaccine products. But the achievement of immunization goals requires more than the discovery of a vaccine. A complex web of financial and institutional arrangements representing a unique public and private partnership is involved in moving a vaccine from the product discovery phase, through the production and development cycle, to licensing and recommendation for general or specialized use, and into the health care delivery system. This partnership is

---

[4]Data for 1999 indicate that 31.9 percent of this high-risk population had received annual influenza vaccinations, while only 17.1 percent had ever received a pneumococcal vaccination (National Center for Health Statistics [NCHS], 2000).

characterized by an array of objectives and incentives that push and pull various components of the immunization process in different directions.

The Societal Benefits of Vaccines

The development of vaccines represents one of the top ten public health achievements of the 20th century (Orenstein, 2002a). The health benefits of vaccines, represented by the protection they confer against infectious disease, accrue not only to the individual who receives the vaccines but also to other members of the community. Benefits to the community accrue because immunization interrupts the transmission of infectious disease by reducing the number of persons who are capable of spreading the infection, as well as the expenses associated with treatment of the disease, especially in public health facilities. Even though some individuals may not be immunized, the presence of high numbers of immunized persons within a community can interrupt and reduce the transmission of vaccine-preventable disease, a process known as "herd immunity." Herd immunity protects those who cannot receive the vaccine because of medical conditions, those who may be too young to receive the vaccine, and those who are not vaccinated because of parental indifference or religious or philosophical objections to vaccination. In addition, immunization benefits families (who are relieved of the burden of care for ill members) and employers (who must replace workers who need to care for ill dependents or who become ill themselves).

The costs and benefits of individual vaccines vary with the type of disease burden and costs associated with each product and with the assumptions that guide the assessment of financial and social benefits. Some vaccines produce significant benefits in early childhood; others provide protection during adolescence or adult life. The benefits of some vaccines are associated with their impact on mortality due to life-threatening diseases (such as measles); others (such as varicella or pneumococcal conjugate) are beneficial because they reduce the burden of illness or morbidity. Some vaccines are recommended for universal use; others are recommended only for certain jurisdictions or populations that have specific risk characteristics. Factors such as cost, protective efficacy, disease incidence, and disease outcomes determine the value of each vaccine.

Considerable research has been devoted to quantifying the specific value and effects of vaccines, for both vaccines currently available and those yet to be developed (IOM, 2000b). Comparing the benefit–cost ratios of different vaccines is difficult, however. Certain vaccines will rank higher than others if calculations are performed solely according to cost per life-year saved (see Table 1-2). Ratios of vaccination benefits to costs can vary substantially, from 27:1 for diphtheria/pertussis (i.e., $27 worth

TABLE 1-2 Benefit–Cost Ratios for Selected Vaccines

Vaccine	Benefit–Cost Ratio (in dollars)	Source
DTaP	27.00: 1	Ekwueme et al., 2000
Hib	5.4: 1	Zhou et al., 2002
MMR	23.3: 1	Zhou et al., in press
Polio (inactivated polio virus [IPV])	5.45: 1	Zhou[a]
Perinatal hepatitis B	14.70: 1	Zhou[a]
Varicella	5.40: 1	Lieu et al., 1994a
Varicella	5.61: 1	Jacobs and Meyerhoff, 2001[b]
Varicella	4.76: 1	Jacobs and Meyerhoff, 2001[c]
Hepatitis A	1.96: 1	Jacobs and Meyerhoff, 2001
Pneumococcal conjugate	0.68: 1	Jacobs and Meyerhoff, 2001
Pneumococcal conjugate	1.1: 1	Derived by CDC from Lieu et al., 2000a (CDC, 2003c)

[a]Personal communication from F. Zhou, March, 2003.
[b]Based on analysis in Huse et al., 1994.
[c]Based on analysis in Preblud et al., 1986.
NOTES: Three methods were used in the analyses:
(1) Single birth cohort, using pre- and postvaccination surveillance data: DTaP, Hib, MMR, polio (IPV); (2) Single birth cohort, using vaccine efficacy: perinatal hepatitis B, varicella (Huse),[b] varicella (Preblud),[c] hepatitis A, and pneumococcal conjugate; (3) Multiple cohorts, dynamic model, using vaccine efficacy: varicella (Lieu et al., 1994a)
SOURCES: CDC and published reports as noted.

of benefits for every $1 spent), to 13.5:1 for measles, 4.76:1 for varicella, and 0.68:1–1.1:1 for pneumococcal conjugate (CDC, 2003c) (see Table 1-2). Such ratios can underrepresent a vaccine's value, however. Additional benefits gained from vaccines, some of which were noted above, include reductions in lost work time, enhanced productivity, increased school attendance, and mitigation of pain and suffering—most of which have not yet become standard elements of vaccine cost–benefit analysis (Lieu et al., 2000a). It should be noted that the benefits of interest here are public health benefits and do not include special considerations associated with national emergencies.

The personal and societal health benefits of vaccines form the foundation for their unique status in the health care system. School children are required to demonstrate proof of immunization prior to school enrollment. Similar requirements are frequently in place for child care centers, nursing homes, and occupational settings such as hospitals and other health care centers. These requirements essentially form a government mandate for vaccines, administered by the states but informed by the recommendations of ACIP, the American Academy of Pediatrics (AAP), and the American Academy of Family Physicians (AAFP).

Vaccine Pricing Trends

Many vaccines with high societal benefit have traditionally been available at low prices. In the 1980s, for example, vaccines such as diphtheria–tetanus–whole-cell pertussis (DTP), oral poliovirus (OPV), and measles–mumps–rubella (MMR) were frequently priced below $3 per dose and in some cases were available for pennies (see Table 1-3). By 2000, however, the prices of newer and improved vaccines for the same diseases had risen significantly. Furthermore, recent additions to the immunization schedule—such as varicella and pneumococcal conjugate—have been priced at substantially higher levels (Table 1-4). The four-dose series of the pneumococcal conjugate vaccine, for example, is priced at $235 (CDC, 2003d).

As a result of these trends, the price of acquiring the full series of recommended immunizations for 2-year-old children in 2002 was $432, more than double the price of complying with the recommended series in 1999 (Davis et al., 2002) (see Figure 1-1). And the prices of future vaccines that are in the early stages of development can be expected to be higher still. The estimated prices of the candidate vaccines reviewed in the IOM

TABLE 1-3 Prices of Selected U.S. Vaccines: 1980 Versus 2003 (U.S. $ per dose)

Year/Product	Public Sector	Private Sector
1980		
Diphtheria–tetanus–whole-cell pertussis (DTP)	0.15	0.30
Oral poliovirus (OPV)	0.35	1.60
Measles–mumps–rubella (MMR)	2.71	7.24
2003		
Diphtheria–tetanus–acellular pertussis (DTaP)	11.75	19.65
Inactivated poliovirus (IPV)	8.80	22.53
Measles–mumps–rubella (MMR)	15.64	34.73
Varicella	41.44	58.11

SOURCES: Personal communication with B. Snyder, Centers for Disease Control and Prevention, 2001; CDC, 2003d.

TABLE 1-4 Vaccines for Children Program: CDC Vaccine Price List (prices as of March 4, 2003)

Vaccine	Manufacturer	Brandname/ Trade name	CDC Cost/ Dose	Private- Sector Cost/Dose
DTaP[a,b]	Aventis Pasteur	Tripedia® DAPTACEL®	$11.75 to $12.75	$19.65 to $20.24
DTaP[a,b]	GlaxoSmithKline	Infanrix®	$11.75 to $12.00	$19.65
DTaP–Hep B–IPV	GlaxoSmithKline	Pediarix	$32.75	$60.06
DTaP–Hib[b,c]	Aventis Pateur	TriHIBit®	$23.40	$38.21
e-IPV[a,d]	Aventis Pasteur	IPOL®	$8.80	$22.53 to $23.31
Hepatitis B– Hib[b,e]	Merck	COMVAX®	$21.83	$43.56
Hepatitis A- Pediatric[b]	Merck	VAQTA®	$11.15	$29.62
Hepatitis A- Pediatric[b]	GlaxoSmithKline	Havrix®	$11.15 to $11.40	$29.73
Hepatitis A- Adult[b]	Merck	VAQTA®	$17.75	$29.62
Hepatitis A- Adult[b]	GlaxoSmithKline	Havrix®	$16.51 to $17.75	$59.45
Hepatitis A– Hepatitis B- 18 only[b,d]	GlaxoSmithKline	Twinrix®	$36.16	$78.67
Hepatitis A– Hepatitis B Adult[b,d]	GlaxoSmithKline	Twinrix®	$36.16	$77.67
Hepatitis B[b,d] Pediatric/ Adolescent	GlaxoSmithKline	ENGERIX B®	$9.00 to $9.25	$24.20
Hepatitis B[b,d] Pediatric/ Adolescent	Merck	RECOMBIVAX HB®	$9.00	$23.20

TABLE 1-4 Continued

Vaccine	Manufacturer	Brandname/ Trade name	CDC Cost/ Dose	Private- Sector Cost/Dose
Hepatitis B- 2 dosed Adolescent (11–15)	Merck	RECOMBIVAX HB®	$24.25	$59.09
Hepatitis B- Adult[b,d]	Merck	RECOMBIVAX HB®	$24.25	$59.09
Hepatitis B- Adult[b,d]	GlaxoSmithKline	ENGERIX-B®	$24.25	$51.73
Hib[b,d]	Merck	PedvaxHIB®	$8.32	$21.52
Hib[b,d]	Wyeth/Lederle	HibTITER®	$7.33	$15.88
Hib[b,d]	Aventis Pasteur	ActHIB®	$7.51	$21.78
Influenza	Aventis Pasteur	Fluzone	$5.525	$6.50
MMR[a,b]	Merck	MMRII®	$15.64	$34.73
Pneumococcal 7-valent[b,d] (Pediatric)	Wyeth/Lederle	Prevnar®	$45.99	$58.75
Rubella[b,d]	Merck	Meuvax II®	$6.54	$14.24
Varicella[b,d]	Merck	Varivax®	$41.44	$58.11

[a]Vaccine cost includes $2.25/dose federal excise tax.
[b]Vaccines that do not contain thimerosal as a preservative.
[c]Vaccine cost includes $3.00/dose federal excise tax.
[d]Vaccine cost includes $0.75/dose federal excise tax.
[e]Vaccine cost includes $1.50/dose federal excise tax.

SOURCE: CDC, 2003d.

report *Vaccines for the 21st Century* (IOM, 2000b), for example, range between $50 and $500 per dose.

The higher prices of new vaccine products have a significant impact on federal budgets designed for the purchase of vaccines for disadvantaged populations. Vaccine suppliers need to negotiate their prices with

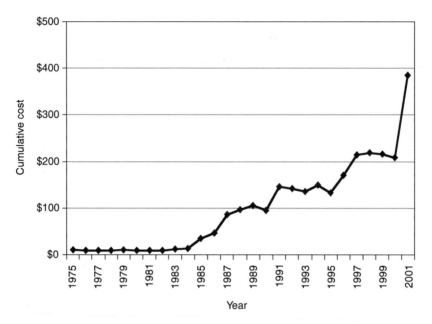

FIGURE 1-1 Cumulative vaccine cost trends.
SOURCE: Davis et al., 2002.

CDC, which purchases over half the volume of vaccines distributed in the United States. Parents and/or their insurance plan must also buy vaccines for their children or themselves. As noted earlier, government establishes a mandate for vaccine use and assists some, but not all, populations in gaining access to the vaccines necessary to fulfill that mandate.

Negotiating on behalf of state as well as federal purchasers, CDC is in the conflicted position of both promoting the development of methods to fight disease (including the use of vaccines) and seeking to keep purchase prices as low as possible (McGuire, 2003). CDC has used its monopsonistic purchasing power to "insist" on lower prices for new vaccines (Miller, 2002).[5] In the case of older vaccines (such as diphtheria–tetanus–acellular pertussis [DTaP] and MMR), federal price caps have been established through legislative action, most notably within the Vaccines for Children (VFC) entitlement.

---

[5]A monopsony is a market situation in which a single purchaser exerts a disproportionate influence on the market.

The tension between the need to establish low prices for public purchases of vaccines and the need to sustain a vigorous vaccine industry is troubling. The prices paid for vaccines now will influence future investments in new products insofar as the current prices affect firms' expectations about profits to be derived through future prices for vaccines under development (McGuire, 2003). Some observers have argued that present pricing policies diminish the incentives to invest in vaccine development and production capacity (Rappuoli et al., 2002). According to this view, the social value of vaccine development is very high relative to vaccine prices, and policies that reduce profits to achieve a vaccine at lower prices are shortsighted (McGuire, 2003).

Assurance and Availability of Vaccines

The development of vaccines and recognition of their social value are fundamental in constructing a successful immunization system but are not sufficient alone to assure that vaccines will be available to all who need them. Vaccines are administered to children and adults in the United States through a public and private health care system that consists of multiple components, including clinicians, insurers, health clinics, employer health programs, and stand-alone immunization events that may occur in schools or other community centers. Each component plays an important role in purchasing, storing, distributing, and administering vaccines to children and adults. Together they form a multifaceted system that is responsible for administering almost a dozen vaccines to an annual birth cohort of more than 4 million children, including more than 11,000 children who are born each day (IOM, 2000a). The immunization system also addresses the vaccination needs of adolescents and adults, a role that involves fewer vaccines, longer time periods between the administration of vaccines, and greater emphasis on targeting vaccines toward at-risk populations.

The total cost of purchasing vaccines for the recommended childhood schedule for children up to age 2 is currently about $400 (this figure includes only the vaccine product cost and does not cover the vaccine administration fee commonly charged by clinicians) (CDC, 2003c,d). Some individuals receive vaccines free of charge because preventive care (including immunizations) is covered by their private health care plan. Others receive vaccines without charge because they are enrolled in a government-supported Medicaid program or State Children's Health Insurance Program (SCHIP). Some insured individuals must pay for their vaccines, even though they have private insurance, if their health plan does not cover vaccines or has a deductible and/or copayments for such services; these individuals are referred to as the *underinsured.*[6] Some states use state revenues to support a universal purchase arrangement that covers vaccinations whether the individual has private insurance or not.

For the clinicians who administer vaccines, these differences can involve serious financial exposure, causing some private practices to refer patients to public health clinics for immunization services. The process of determining eligibility for vaccination and the disparities involved in payment arrangements are attracting increasing attention in the health care system. The complexity of the nature and scope of different purchasing arrangements and immunization practices is a major challenge to the task of examining how the costs of immunization are distributed across public and private health care systems.

This study examines two key goals of the national immunization system and considers their relationship to vaccine finance arrangements:

- *Assurance.* Assuring access to vaccines for all those who need them is a fundamental goal of the public health system. Assuring access involves certain key considerations, such as the cost, coverage, and distribution of immunization resources. Over the past decade, the role of public health agencies has shifted from one of providing direct access to vaccines in public health clinics to one of assuring that vaccines are covered within public and private health plans, especially those that serve disadvantaged populations.
- *Availability.* Assuring access to vaccines is of little use if the vaccine supply and delivery system is disrupted or if clinicians are not able to provide vaccines to patients because of financial considerations. Therefore, this study examines the many factors that influence the use of vaccines in routine health care interactions. Similarly, the goal of assuring that a reliable vaccine supply system is in place requires examination of the incentives that influence investments in vaccine production and development.

Over time, the interactions between the goals of assurance and availability have become increasingly complex. The effort to integrate the immunization process directly into the delivery of routine health care services has fostered the development of myriad programs and safety net services designed to assure that all children have access to recommended

---

[6]This report follows the CDC National Immunization Program's definition of *underinsured*, which includes only those persons who have medical insurance coverage that excludes coverage for immunizations. This definition does not encompass the additional population of individuals who have insurance with high deductibles and copayments, even if these costs limit their access to vaccines.

vaccines regardless of their income level or location. Yet efforts to reduce or contain the costs of these programs have raised fundamental concerns about the extent to which private clinicians and vaccine suppliers will be able to continue their participation in the vaccine supply and system.

Initial warning signs of increased tensions have already appeared in the form of delays in reimbursement to health care providers for vaccine costs, shortages in the vaccine supply system, dwindling numbers of vaccine manufacturers in the United States, gaps in the coverage of recommended vaccines by private health plans, and hesitation to recommend newly licensed vaccines because of concerns about higher costs. The fact that at least six of the routine childhood vaccines, as well as the adult influenza vaccine, are produced by foreign manufacturers has been raised as an additional concern. Before these tensions reach crisis proportions, it is appropriate to step back and assess whether public resources are being employed wisely. In particular, this study examines whether the strategies and finance arrangements that have evolved over the past few decades are sufficient to address the burden of an accelerating number of new vaccine products for diverse child and adult populations in the future.

STUDY PROCESS

The IOM formed the Committee on the Evaluation of Vaccine Purchase Financing in the United States in 2002 to carry out this study. The 11-member committee[7] met four times within a 12-month period, receiving expert testimony and the perspectives of representatives of CDC, the vaccine industry, and public and private health plans, as well as employee benefit managers and clinicians. The committee commissioned a national survey and eight background papers to inform its discussions (see Appendices C and D, respectively, for descriptions of the survey and the commissioned papers). Further analyses and data were provided by CDC's National Immunization Program, a survey of health plans conducted by the American Association of Health Plans (AAHP, 2002), and data obtained with the assistance of the American Medical Group Association from individual member groups. The committee also received materials from four companies that distribute childhood vaccines in the United States (Aventis Pasteur, GlaxoSmithKline, Merck, and Wyeth-Lederle). Although the committee requested industry data on vaccine

---

[7]Biographies of the committee members are provided in Appendix E. A twelfth committee member, Sam Ho, attended no committee meetings and resigned in August 2002.

pricing, distribution, production, and profits, it was unable to obtain access to primary data or proprietary information.

The committee also benefited from a series of earlier IOM studies on vaccine finance and vaccine policy issues (IOM, 1985, 1993, 1995, 2000a,b).[8] A series of IOM workshop reports on immunization finance further informed the committee's discussions (IOM, 2002a,b, 2003).

Several key reports published during the study period provided additional perspective and data sources. These included a report by the General Accounting Office (GAO) (2002) on vaccine supply, a report on vaccine supply issues prepared by the National Vaccine Advisory Committee (NVAC, 2003), and a report prepared for the Global Alliance for Vaccines Initiative (Mercer Management Consulting, 2002). The IOM report on *The Future of Public's Health in the 21st Century* (IOM, 2002c) also informed the committee's deliberations.

SUMMING UP

Despite the improvements in child and adult immunization rates over the past decade, troubling signs persist in the form of the differences between public health goals and actual rates of immunization, disparities in state-level and urban rates, and the burden of vaccine-preventable disease among the elderly and high-risk adult populations. In addition, tensions have emerged in both assuring access to vaccines and sustaining the availability of a reliable supply of vaccines in the health care system during periods of fiscal restraint and higher prices for new vaccine products. Health officials have expressed concern that higher costs will lead to reduced health plan benefits for immunization and that low administration fees and the burden associated with checking the status of vaccine benefits are contributing to missed opportunities and private-sector referrals to public health clinics. The result will be lower rates of immunization, greater disparities in immunization rates, and possible outbreaks of vaccine-preventable disease.

Any one of the challenges discussed above could have a profound impact on immunization. Combined, they contribute to a sense of urgency about the long-term viability of the public–private partnership that supports the national immunization system. The purpose of this study was to consider what is known about the experience with existing vaccine purchase programs. Building on this knowledge base, the committee sought

---

[8]The Institute of Medicine has also published more than a dozen studies on topics related to vaccine safety and military issues that are not cited here.

to develop a long-term finance strategy that can achieve the goals of assuring access to recommended vaccines in the settings where children and adults receive routine health care, as well as creating incentives to sustain a reliable and innovative supply of vaccines now and in the decades ahead.

Public concern about fair access, low costs, and a reliable and innovative vaccine supply has stimulated many proposals for reform in vaccine payment, pricing, regulatory, patent, stockpile, and health insurance systems (Fairbrother and Haidery, 2002). The interaction of policy objectives suggests that no single approach is sufficient to address all significant concerns. The evidentiary base associated with selected reforms in vaccine financing and delivery is not well developed, and uncertainty pervades the decision-making process. Yet to do nothing at this juncture because of the complexity of the problem could result in a further reduction in access to vaccines and discourage the development of effective new vaccines.

ORGANIZATION OF THE REPORT

The remainder of this report consists of six chapters. Chapter 2 provides a historical overview of the origins and rationale of the U.S. immunization system and describes the different federal, state, and private components that shape national vaccine policy. Chapter 3 describes aspects of vaccine finance related to public and private insurance coverage, including private health care plans and such public plans as Medicare, Medicaid, VFC, and SCHIP. Chapter 4 focuses on the health care delivery system, examining arrangements for clinician reimbursement and factors that influence access to vaccines in routine health care settings. Chapter 5 addresses what is known about vaccine availability by highlighting key aspects of the vaccine supply system. This chapter provides a broad overview of the role of private industry in producing and distributing vaccines to public and private health care providers, as well as the role of the governmental contracting process in establishing vaccine prices for public-sector purchase. Chapter 6 presents the committee's conclusions, as well as alternative vaccine finance strategies considered for this study. The committee's recommendations are given in Chapter 7.

Origins and Rationale of Immunization Policy
Summary of Findings

- Government is deeply involved in the immunization enterprise, a role that reflects the public-good and spillover characteristics of vaccines.
- Government policy toward vaccine research and development (R&D) is inconsistent: it both promotes and discourages the development of new vaccines.
- While states continue to take principal responsibility for immunization infrastructure and delivery, it can no longer be assumed that they will share responsibility for vaccine purchase with the federal government.
- It cannot be assumed that private insurers will continue to share responsibility for covering immunizations.
- The assumption of a stable supply of vaccines produced by a healthy private sector can no longer be made.
- The current approaches to vaccine prioritization and immunization system planning are inadequate, as currently structured, to deal with the changing nature of vaccines and vaccine economics.

2

Origins and Rationale of Immunization Policy

The national immunization system is the culmination of public health legislation and traditions dating to the early 1800s, which include the participation of state and federal governments as well as the private sector. The immunization system today benefits from substantial government support, including federal support for basic research and development (R&D) through the National Institutes of Health (NIH); federal and state funding for public health outreach, infrastructure development, and vaccine purchase; and regulation of the quality of vaccines through the Food and Drug Administration (FDA) (see Table 2-1).

Government also supports vaccination in some special ways. For example, state governments mandate and enforce immunization through school entry requirements, and a few WIC agencies ask parents to pick up food stamps more frequently until their children are up to date on immunizations. With the passage of the Vaccines for Children (VFC) program in 1993, Congress enacted a major new federal health care entitlement. This program guarantees federally purchased vaccines to more than 10 million children nationwide[1] (Wood, 2003). More than 14 states now have universal immunization programs that provide all or most vaccines to every child in the state, regardless of insurance coverage (Freed and Cowan, 2002). (State financing systems are listed in Table 3-3 in Chapter 3.)

---

[1]Eligible populations include children in Medicaid, uninsured children aged 18 and under, Native Americans and Alaska Natives, and all children vaccinated in federally qualified health centers (FQHCs).

TABLE 2-1 Government Roles in Immunization

Government Role	Functions	Agency/Program
Supporting R&D	Basic research programs, support of clinical trials	NIH, National Institute for Allergy and Infectious Disease (NIAID)
Regulating safety	Vaccine approval	FDA Center for Biologics Evaluation and Research (CBER)
	Safety monitoring	CDC Vaccine Adverse Events Reporting System (VAERS), CDC Vaccine Safety DataLink
Promoting, monitoring, and enforcing immunization	Recommending the vaccine schedule	Advisory Committee on Immunization Practices (ACIP)
	Monitoring	CDC disease surveillance, CDC National Immunization Survey (NIS), CDC grantee reporting and evaluation process, registries
	Enforcement	State school entry laws, state nursing home requirements, state child day care requirements, travel requirements
Purchasing vaccines	Direct federal purchase	VFC, Veterans Administration, Department of Defense/ CHAMPUS
	Grants to states	CDC Section 317 grants to states
	State purchase	State employee coverage, universal purchase programs, other state purchases
Promoting and regulating adequate vaccine supply	Stockpiles	National stockpile program
	Coordination	Linking producers, state health officials, providers, CDC
	Protecting suppliers from liability	National Vaccine Injury Compensation Fund
	Government production	Massachusetts vaccine production program

TABLE 2-1 Continued

Government Role	Functions	Agency/Program
Infrastructure development	Direct investment in and operation of public health delivery systems	States, CDC Section 317 grants to states
	Setting reimbursement rates for vaccines and administration fees	Medicare Resource-Based Relative Value Scale (RBRVS) rates, state Medicaid programs
	Supporting registry development	CDC Section 317 program
	Supporting state universal purchase programs	CDC
	Establishing physician participation in Medicaid/VFC	CDC
Regulating insurance coverage	VFC maintenance-of-effort law	CDC/states
	State insurance requirements	States

The federal government uses its substantial purchasing power to negotiate discounted vaccine prices for these federal and state programs. Between VFC, the Veterans Administration, the Department of Defense, and state governments, the public sector purchases the majority of vaccines sold in the United States.

This deep public involvement in the national immunization system is based in part on the public-good properties and spillover effects that characterize vaccines (see Box 2-1). Because of these properties, the enormous benefits of vaccines are likely to be undervalued by society, and both the rates of immunization by the public sector and the levels of private investment in new vaccine R&D are likely to be lower than desirable without additional incentives. At the same time, these properties of vaccines make the case for public support of immunization very strong. This support is reflected in federal and state programs designed to encourage immunization, such as VFC and CDC Section 317 grants to states. It also includes inducements to industry, through the patent system, to invest in production and research. Government policy regarding stimulation of vaccine R&D, however, is inconsistent. While the government encourages such investment through the patent system, it also discourages that same investment by using its purchasing leverage, its legislative power, and the imposition of price caps to secure substantial price discounts for existing vaccines.

BOX 2-1
Vaccine Spillover Effects and Public Good Properties

Vaccines occupy a unique place in health care policy because of their *spillover effects,* or *positive consumption externalities,* and their *public-good* characteristics. Both of these concepts influenced the committee's analysis.

Positive consumption externalities or **spillover effects** exist when consumption of a product by one person benefits both the individual who consumes it and others who do not consume it. Vaccines against highly contagious infectious diseases have strong spillover effects, since immunization protects not just those being immunized but others as well. Since the benefits extend beyond those individuals who choose to get vaccinated, the public benefits of vaccines are much larger than the individual benefits. The price will reflect only the private benefit—what individuals are willing to pay to protect themselves. As a result, expenditures on vaccines will be smaller than if the price incorporated the benefits to society as a whole. To remedy this problem, government could subsidize the positive externality to force consumers to act as if they internalized the external effects. Public health strategies might include charging less than the market price for vaccines, paying individuals to immunize, or making immunization compulsory.

Differences in Spillover Effects Among Vaccines. Some vaccines protect against highly contagious infectious diseases, while others protect against infectious diseases that are not easily transmitted from one person to another. Measles is highly contagious, and therefore the measles vaccine has strong spillover effects. The vaccine for tetanus, a disease typically contracted through injuries, does not have such properties. In this regard, the tetanus vaccine is similar to other preventive services, such as mammograms or colonoscopies. A number of the vaccines now in development, such as therapeutic vaccines for arthritis, diabetes, and cancer, fit into this nonspillover category. Vaccines that are targeted to high-risk groups (e.g., immuno-compromised adults at risk for pneumonia and those at behavioral risk for HIV) rather than to the general population fall into a gray area. While they afford some protection to the public at large, they confer substantially higher benefits to those who are at higher risk and this supports the development of a private market.

Other Interventions with Spillover Effects. Once someone has contracted an infectious disease, treatment can also have spillover effects. By taking an antibiotic that suppresses and eliminates a contagious disease, the individual prevents further transmission to others. The main difference is that once someone has contracted a disease, a strong private motive exists for seeking treatment. Thus private markets may be adequate to achieve social goals without additional subsidies.

Comparison with Public Goods. A **public good** is a product whose benefits extend to all people at no greater cost than that to provide it for one person. The benefits of the product are indivisible, and no one can be excluded from using it. For example, national defense is considered a public good because it benefits everyone and can exclude no one. In this way, a public good contrasts with a private good, such as bread, which if consumed by one person cannot be consumed by another.

Vaccine research and development has public-good properties because it involves the identification of basic scientific knowledge that benefits everyone and is not diminished by someone's use of that knowledge. Two individuals may not take the same dose of a vaccine, but they both can benefit from the same knowledge that led to the production of the vaccine. Vaccines are not unique in this property; it can apply in varying degrees to many socially beneficial goods, such as medical research, technology, books, and even ideas.

Public goods provide an important rationale for government intervention. Because public goods cannot be divided and sold to the individuals they benefit, private markets for such goods are sometimes difficult to develop. In the absence of patent or copyright protection, the market is frequently not able to provide such goods and services unless property rights are granted or adequate alternative compensation is available through other mechanisms, such as taxes. In public policy debate, public-good properties can be ascribed to many aspects of health care, such as health insurance for the poor.

Confusion with "Social Goods." A product that offers extremely high benefits to society is not necessarily a public good, nor does it necessarily have spillover effects. A drug that controls cholesterol and prevents heart attacks is clearly a social good, but it is not a public good; it benefits primarily the person taking it, resulting in a private market for the product. It has limited spillover effects, because it benefits primarily the person taking the drug and provides no benefit to others at risk of the disease.

continued

BOX 2-1 Continued

Type of Product	Definition	Examples
Spillover effects or positive consumption externalities	When consumption of a product by one person benefits others, the spillover effects or positive consumption externalities are the benefits that accrue to those who do not consume it.	• Measles vaccine • Influenza vaccine • Pertussis vaccine • To a lesser extent, antibiotics
Public good	A product whose benefits may be provided to all people at no greater cost than that to provide it for one person. The benefits of the product are indivisible, and people cannot be excluded from using it.	• National defense • Vaccine research and development (has public-good properties because the underlying scientific knowledge is not diminished by individual consumption) • Medical knowledge
Private good	A good that, if consumed by one person, cannot be consumed by another.	• Bread • Prescription drugs, other than anti-infectives • Tetanus vaccine • Diabetes vaccine (in development) • Cancer vaccines (in development)
Social good	A product that offers extremely high benefits to society; it may or may not be a public good.	• All of the above

The compelling public interest in a strong and effective vaccine system has been well served by the national immunization system. But the assumptions and traditions guiding immunization policy have changed, and the worsening economic landscape has put additional pressure on the system. It is unlikely that this system can effectively serve the public in the future without undergoing substantial change. As context for the remainder of the report, this chapter examines the legislative origins of the current system, explains the shared federal and state responsibility for financing of vaccine purchases and the shared public and private responsibility for immunization coverage, describes public and private immunization delivery systems, reviews private vaccine production, and summarizes the process used for setting national vaccine policy.

LEGISLATIVE HISTORY OF VACCINE POLICY

The historical roots of the current U.S. immunization system reside in a federal–state–private-sector partnership that has evolved through a series of responses to infectious disease crises.[2] Although the scale of effort has expanded significantly over the past 50 years, the federal government's role remained relatively unchanged from the mid-1950s to the early 1990s.

The earliest federal legislation pertaining to vaccines was the Virus Serums and Toxins Act, passed by Congress in 1902 "to regulate the sale of viruses, serums, toxins, and analogues productions…" in interstate and foreign commerce. The laboratory of the Public Health Service was subsequently authorized to conduct inspections and to ensure the safety of vaccine products. The regulatory authority for both of these functions was eventually transferred to NIH in 1948 and in 1972 was transferred again to FDA.

In addition to its regulatory and licensing role, the federal government has provided financial support to state and local health departments for maternal and child health programs since the 1920s (Orenstein et al., 1999). These programs, funded by block grants authorized under Title V of the Social Security Act, represent a federal–state partnership that has been in place for more than 60 years. Title V embedded immunization services into a comprehensive safety net system for children and their

---

[2]Much of the descriptive information in this section is taken from Johnson et al. (2000). See also Fee and Brown (2002) and Lumpkin and Richards (2002) for discussions of the history and future of public health. Orenstein et al. (1999) provide a good overview of the immunization system.

mothers. When the polio vaccine was licensed, Congress quickly passed the Poliomyelitis Immunization Assistance Act of 1955 to expedite the state purchase of vaccine for susceptible children and pregnant women by circumventing the ponderous Maternal and Child Health grant process. A total of $53.6 million was appropriated in 1956 and 1957 for state purchase of vaccines (Freeman and Robbins, 1991).

The successful effort to halt polio epidemics stimulated interest in identifying opportunities to prevent other childhood diseases. In the early 1960s, the Kennedy Administration launched the Immunization Assistance Act of 1962, which provided federal support to state and local immunization programs using oral polio vaccines, as well as diphtheria, pertussis, and tetanus (DPT) vaccines. The legislation established a federal presence in the financing of childhood vaccines but not direct purchase.

Beginning in 1965, substantial changes occurred in federal immunization policy that continued over the next decade. The first bulk purchases of vaccines under a federal contract occurred in fiscal year 1966, when the federal government purchased polio and measles vaccines under consolidated contracts and provided them in lieu of financial grants to state and local public health agencies. The purpose of this policy change was to offset the costs incurred by state and local public health agencies, since the bulk purchase of vaccines under a federal contract led to substantial price reductions. Additional vaccines, including the rubella and combined measles–mumps–rubella (MMR) vaccines, were added to the federal vaccine contract between 1969 and 1975. Even as late as 1982, however, diphtheria and tetanus toxoids and whole-cell pertussis (DTP) vaccines were not being purchased under the federal contract because their prices were low, and limited savings could be achieved by bulk purchases. In addition, Congress enacted Section 317 of the Public Health Service Act in 1972 to provide grants to state and local governments for immunization infrastructure development and vaccine purchases.

By the late 1980s, childhood immunization rates had achieved record highs. Nevertheless, measles outbreaks occurred in several parts of the United States during 1989 and 1990, catching public health officials off guard. The outbreaks resulted in over 55,000 cases of measles, 130 deaths, 11,000 hospitalizations and 44,000 hospital days, and an estimated $150 million in direct medical costs (Shalala, 1993). The traditional shared federal–state responsibility for infectious disease control was challenged by the variability of state efforts and the inability of states to marshal sufficient funding to respond to the outbreaks. Increased federal funds became available to fill the gaps, and the Department of Health and Human Services (DHHS) undertook a study of federal and state acquisition and reimbursement policies for vaccines (Kelly et al., 1993). The study identified systematic barriers to access as the key limiting factor for immunization rates and suggested the elimination of fragmentation and conflicting rules among government programs.

In 1994, the VFC program was launched as part of national health care reform efforts during the Clinton Administration. The centerpiece of the program is an entitlement that provides free vaccines to children aged 18 and younger who are uninsured, Alaska Native or Native American, or who eligible for Medicaid, or receive their vaccines in a federally qualified health center (FQHC). A key goal of the program is to enable children receiving public assistance to be immunized within their medical home rather than in a public health clinic. The result has been a massive shift of safety net immunizations from approximately 3,300 public clinics to well over 40,000 private providers. This program has also expanded the public share of vaccine purchases from roughly 35 percent to 52–55 percent of all childhood vaccines (Orenstein, 2002a). Under the program, CDC negotiates the prices of vaccines, which are then ordered by the states at the federal contract price.

Today the federal government is active in virtually every aspect of immunization—from basic research to the purchase of vaccines (Schwartz and Orenstein, 2001). The National Institute of Allergy and Infectious Diseases (NIAID) within NIH supports basic research and clinical trials. Safety and efficacy are regulated by FDA's Center for Biologics Evaluation and Research (CBER), which reviews new vaccine applications; reviews clinical trials; and licenses new vaccines, production facilities, and each lot of vaccine that is produced. Postrelease safety is monitored through the CDC Vaccine Adverse Event Reporting System (VAERS) and the Vaccine Safety DataLink (VSD). VSD is a CDC program in which eight health maintenance organizations (HMOs) across the United States combine data on immunizations so that potential rare adverse events that may be associated with some vaccines can be identified and evaluated.

CDC also monitors immunization rates through its annual National Immunization Survey, conducts ongoing disease surveillance, and monitors state and metropolitan grantees. CDC negotiates federal contracts for the public purchase of vaccines for the VFC program and state purchase, which account for more than half of childhood vaccines sold in the United States. CDC also determines Section 317 funding to state grantees, maintains the national vaccine stockpile, and supports state immunization program offices.

SHARED FEDERAL AND STATE
RESPONSIBILITY FOR FINANCING

Despite the deep federal involvement in immunization, states and localities retain primary responsibility for providing public health services, including the maintenance of a public health infrastructure. States develop and fund a public vaccine delivery system—including facilities, equipment, drugs and supplies, health professionals, and administration—that provides a broad safety net for the underserved. States are largely responsible for enforcement of immunization through school entry, nursing home, and day care laws. Many states maintain or are developing a statewide registry to track both immunization status and eligibility. States also enforce mandates for state-regulated health insurance plans, although this responsibility excludes self-insured employer plans that are exempt under the Employee Retirement and Income Security Act (ERISA). In addition, states conduct continuous outbreak surveillance, maintain registries, pay providers, carry out planning activities, forecast vaccine demand, and perform public outreach.

States rely heavily on federal assistance to maintain this delivery infrastructure. The Section 317 program provides grants to states for both vaccine purchase and infrastructure. The national immunization system has historically been based on an assumption of shared federal and state responsibility for immunization financing. Over the last decade, however, the state role in financing immunization has waned. Today, fewer than half of the states contribute more than 10 percent of government vaccine expenditures, and only 10 states contribute more than half (Federal Funds Information for States, 2002; Freed and Cowan, 2002). The erosion of the state role accelerated with the passage of the VFC program. VFC was intended to enhance, but not supplant, state funding for immunization; between the introduction of VFC in 1994 and 2002, however, state spending on immunization lagged well behind federal spending. States contributed an estimated $340 million to immunization in fiscal year 2000, of which $109 million was for vaccine purchase (IOM, 2000a).

VFC funding has increased substantially. Many states have allowed these new federal dollars to partially replace (or crowd out) state funds in meeting the state's vaccine needs (Academy for Health Services Research and Health Policy [AHSRHP], 2001). This crowd-out is a natural result of the structure of VFC and state funding streams: as a federal entitlement program, VFC has assured funding, whereas state funding depends upon the discretionary legislative process. The current fiscal crisis in most states exacerbates the pressure for crowd-out.

Despite the general trend toward diminished state support of vaccine purchase, some states have increased their immunization budgets. Starting in the early 1990s, a handful of states established universal purchase programs that use state funds to purchase vaccines for all citizens, regardless of insurance status. Fourteen states now have such programs, although several have excluded the most expensive vaccines. Given the current economic outlook for many states, the expansion of universal purchase programs is unlikely (National Health Policy Forum, 2001).

The long-standing assumption that the federal government and the states will share responsibility for financing of vaccine purchases appears to be challenged, then, by the trends of the past decade. An erosion of shared federal and state responsibility has two potential downsides. First, it reduces the ability of federal and state agencies to distribute the burden of increasing vaccine expenditures and respond to sudden needs or budget shortfalls. Second, the key historical assumption that public health is a state and local activity derives from the need for flexibility and local knowledge and special conditions that defy a one-size-fits-all federal approach. This is particularly true for vaccines because of local conditions that could foster outbreaks, the need for coordinated and interdisciplinary community responses, and concerns regarding public acceptance and enforcement. To the extent that federal vaccine purchasing could limit local flexibility, it might be considered detrimental to public health. In practice, however, increasingly federalized financing for vaccines may have enabled states to focus their resources away from vaccine purchase and toward infrastructure, surveillance, and targeted immunization campaigns. States continue to perform the public health and administrative functions associated with immunization (Freed and Cowan, 2002).

SHARED PUBLIC AND PRIVATE
RESPONSIBILITY FOR COVERAGE

Prior to the last several decades, employer-based private insurance provided limited coverage for preventive services, including immunization. Until recently, the public sector played a highly active role in immunization, particularly during the early polio vaccination campaign of the 1950s. Coverage of preventive services increased, however, with the growth of HMOs, which have traditionally emphasized such services. Eventually, the private sector assumed responsibility for immunizing more than half of the population, and the public role became focused almost exclusively on the safety net function—that is, providing basic health services for underserved and disadvantaged populations. The introduction of the VFC program in 1994 did not fundamentally change this relationship. In fact, a key assumption of the VFC program was that the private sector would continue to share the burden more or less equally with the public sector, and the law included a maintenance-of-effort provision that required private insurers to maintain the childhood immunization benefits they had in place before VFC. In addition, 27 states have imposed separate immunization coverage mandates on state-regulated insurance plans (i.e., excluding self-funded plans exempted from state regulation by ERISA). Eleven states include mandates on adult immunization (Swartz, 2003). There are indications, however, that private insurance coverage of immunization is now eroding:

• Laws designed to prevent such erosion—state mandates and maintenance-of-effort provisions—vary widely in both content and enforcement (Freed and Cowan, 2002; Swartz, 2003). Furthermore, self-insured, ERISA plans are exempt from state laws,[3] and insurance plans instituted since 1994 are exempt from maintenance-of-effort provisions.

• Universal purchase states have shifted from private to public financing as insurers have turned to publicly supplied vaccines for their beneficiaries. In these states, insurers can provide immunization as a covered benefit and then encourage their providers to use VFC vaccines rather than ask for reimbursement for privately purchased vaccines. For example, United Healthcare of Connecticut requires providers to use state-supplied VFC vaccines when they are available (United Healthcare, 2002).

• Coverage tends to vary by type of insurance product, and therefore the mix of insurance products affects coverage levels. HMOs have historically had the highest coverage levels, while preferred provider organizations (PPOs) and indemnity plans provide immunization coverage less frequently (Wood, 2003). Since PPOs are gaining in market share relative to HMOs (Kaiser Family Foundation and Health Research and Educational Trust [KFF-HRET], 2002), average coverage levels may decline.

• Even insurers that provide immunization benefits often require patient cost sharing in the form of deductibles and copayments (KFF-HRET, 2002). The shift in the insurance product mix to PPOs may contribute to this trend.

• Higher vaccine prices may contribute to higher premiums and cause employers or workers to drop health insurance (KFF-HRET, 2002).

These trends in benefits and regulation suggest that underinsurance is a growing problem. Recent surveys indicate that between 5 and 14 percent of insured children do not have coverage for immunizations, and 50 percent of insured adults not on Medicare lack coverage (CDC, 2002d; IOM, 2000a; Meyer, 2002; Wood, 2003). Furthermore, as noted above, many of those who have immunization coverage face significant financial barriers to immunization in the form of cost sharing, such as deductibles

---

[3]For a fuller discussion of applications of ERISA to health benefits, see Butler (2000).

and copayments. Interviews with health plan representatives also suggest that they may rethink the types of vaccine benefits they typically provide for recommended childhood vaccines as newer vaccines with higher prices and less-favorable cost–benefit profiles are developed (Swartz, 2003). Of particular concern to health plans is the development of new and expensive combination vaccines that are likely to be in high demand by parents and providers, although they may not prove to be cost-effective.

What if the assumed shared public and private responsibility for vaccine financing is no longer assured? Sharing the financial burden has been important to states, and its importance increases in tight budgetary environments. Erosion of coverage in a piecemeal fashion could further fragment immunization coverage if, for example, a patient were to have separate providers and funding sources for different vaccines. This fragmentation could lead in turn to missed opportunities and higher administrative costs. On the other hand, public (federal) assumption of all financing responsibility would likely negate these detrimental effects.

PUBLIC AND PRIVATE DELIVERY SYSTEMS

The delivery system for public immunization has experienced major changes during the last decade. Before the adoption of VFC in 1994, patients in Medicaid or other types of public assistance programs usually received vaccines in public health clinics (IOM, 2000a). With VFC, delivery of vaccines for those without insurance shifted from public clinics to private office-based medical practices. This shift aligned immunization services with the two prevailing trends: (1) increasing reliance on private managed care contractors and providers to serve Medicaid and State Children's Health Insurance Program (SCHIP) enrollees, and (2) delivery of safety net services within the "medical home or usual source of care." Thus, VFC expanded the safety net provider base from roughly 3,300 public clinics to more than 40,000 public and private provider sites (IOM, 2000a).

The shift from stand-alone public clinics to office-based, routine sources of care created additional administrative complexity, especially in terms of surveillance: it is more difficult to monitor 40,000 plus provider sites than 3,000 clinics. Furthermore, participating clinicians face administrative burdens as a result of fragmentation that remains within the immunization system. The existence of multiple payors requires determinations of eligibility that can be quite difficult. Ineligibility may result in a provider's not receiving compensation for a vaccine already administered. The combination of VFC and health plan formularies can lead to separate stocks of vaccines and unequal treatment of patients based on source of payment. In addition, problems in the timing of vaccine release and VFC contract negotiations may leave providers with gaps in inventories that result in missed opportunities and high costs associated with patient recall programs. Also, since VFC does not cover clinician fees for administering vaccines, those fees remain even more fragmented than vaccine purchase. These issues contribute to a high rate of referrals of patients to the public sector, even with VFC (Zimmerman et al., 1997).

PRIVATE VACCINE PRODUCTION

Government is not merely a purchaser of vaccines; it works closely with the vaccine industry in several ways. The government supports basic vaccine research through NIH, enforces patent laws that influence the profitability of the industry, regulates the production of vaccines through the FDA, recommends vaccines for the childhood and adult schedules (thereby determining market size and funding streams), and negotiates contracts for more than half of the childhood vaccines purchased in the United States. Massachusetts and Michigan have even engaged in vaccine production. In Box 2-2, public–private collaboration in the supply of vaccines is illustrated through the history of the DTaP vaccine.

The industry–government relationship has for the most part been highly collaborative and constructive, despite normal tensions between a regulator and a regulated entity. Examples of issues that have created tensions include the need for protection from lawsuits over vaccine injury, which resulted in the adoption of the National Vaccine Injury Compensation Program; the removal of thimerosal (a mercury-based preservative) from recommended vaccines; the passage of VFC, which resulted in a larger public share of vaccine purchases and lower average prices; the introduction of the FDA's Team Biologics regulatory regime, which increased the burden of regulatory compliance for producers; the higher industry pricing model for new vaccines, such as varicella and pneumococcal conjugate; unprecedented vaccine shortages; and the increasing burden of proof required for vaccine approval and entry into the U.S. market.

While industry–government conflicts are typically resolved amicably, the changing landscape could exacerbate future conflicts. Given the limited number of vaccine producers left in the market and the risk of even further exit (see Chapter 5), the government has little leverage or room for negotiation on key issues. The increasing number of recommended vaccines and higher prices of new vaccines, along with the changing cost–benefit profiles of newer and combination vaccines, tend to elevate economic considerations and politicize vaccine policy. Most important, these issues increasingly involve government policies that are at cross-purposes. For example, a key approach for alleviating the fragility of supply—

BOX 2-2
Public–Private Collaboration: The Case of DTaP Vaccine

The history of the DTaP vaccine illustrates recent trends in the vaccine industry. DTaP is a combination vaccine that includes diphtheria, tetanus, and acellular pertussis components. Its predecessor, DTP, which used a whole-cell pertussis component, was one of the first combination vaccines to be licensed by the Food and Drug Administration (FDA). DTP was integrated into routine pediatric care in the late 1940s and remained a staple of preventive services in the United States through the mid-1990s (CDC, 1992).

Public Safety

Concerns about the safety of whole-cell pertussis first emerged in the 1930s (Mowery and Mitchell, 1995). Public concern about DTP peaked in Japan and Great Britain in the mid-1970s and led to declines in immunization rates and increases in pertussis cases and deaths in Japan and Great Britain (CDC, 1992; Gangarosa et al., 1998). Researchers in Japan began to search for a more refined, acellular version of the pertussis vaccine (Felton, 1957). In 1981, these efforts paid off with the development of a licensed DTaP vaccine in that country (CDC, 1992; Noble et al., 1987).

The issue peaked in the United States in the early 1980s, in part as a result of television documentaries such as "Vaccine Roulette," which helped sensitize the public and policy makers to vaccine safety concerns. Product-liability lawsuits followed and rapidly escalated—from 17 suits in 1982 to 225 by 1986 (Sing and Willian, 1996). In response to the growing liability crisis, two of the three manufacturers distributing DTP in the U.S. market—Wyeth and Connaught—dropped out in 1984, leaving Lederle as the sole supplier in this country (CDC, 1984). A severe shortage of DTP followed, which necessitated a decision to postpone the fourth and fifth doses, thus assuring coverage for infants, the most vulnerable population (CDC, 1984). In response to the crisis, Congress enacted the National Vaccine Injury Compensation Program (NVICP), a no-fault program to assist victims of vaccine injury, which was funded by a federal excise tax on childhood vaccines (Johnson et al., 2000). The compensation program was effective almost immediately in controlling DTP lawsuits. Congress also established the National Vaccine Program to develop a comprehensive National Vaccine Plan, and established the National Vaccine Advisory Committee to advise the Secretary of Health and Human Services on national vaccine policy.

Research and Development

The development of a licensed acellular pertussis vaccine became a high priority of both the National Institutes of Health (NIH) and the FDA. In addition to conducting basic research (NIH researchers played a key role in the development of the initial acellular pertussis vaccine licensed in Japan in 1981), NIH took an unusually proactive role in financing and

continued

BOX 2-2 Continued

overseeing clinical trials starting in the mid-1980s and continuing into the 1990s. By the late 1990s, four companies had been licensed to manufacture and distribute acellular pertussis products for the U.S. market.

NIH helped accelerate the development and licensing of acellular pertussis vaccines by sponsoring a comprehensive series of clinical trials, which provided a unique opportunity for comparisons across multiple vaccine candidates (National Institutes of Health [NIH], 2002). Starting in 1984, NIH actively and successfully recruited nine manufacturers into Phase II clinical trials, which resulted in a unique collaboration across industry and between industry and government agencies in the United States and abroad (Mowery and Mitchell, 1995). Lederle-Praxis Biologicals took exception to the fact that NIH selected only foreign-made vaccines for the multicenter Phase III trials (Mowery and Mitchell, 1995); but despite its concern, Lederle's DTaP vaccine, Acel-Imune, eventually became the first acellular pertussis vaccine approved for use in the United States (CDC, 1991).

Although the first acellular pertussis vaccines were licensed in Japan in 1981, it would take a full decade, until December 1991, before an acellular pertussis vaccine was approved for American children. This approval was initially only for the fourth and fifth doses; not until 1996 was DTaP approved for the full five-dose series.

Supply

Once DTaP was in production, supplies of the vaccine were stable throughout the 1990s. By 1998, four manufacturers were producing DTaP for the U.S. market. By 1999, 95 percent of U.S. children aged 19–35 months had received three doses and 83 percent had received four doses of DTP or DTaP (CDC, 2000). By January 2001, however, the DTaP supply picture had deteriorated significantly. A nationwide shortage of DTaP led CDC to temporarily revise its recommended childhood immunization schedule (CDC, 2001b; GAO, 2002).

As with other vaccine shortages in 2001–2002, the DTaP shortages have been attributed to multiple factors. The most proximal causes included the abrupt withdrawal from the U.S. market of two manufacturers (Wyeth and North American Vaccine) and a serious slowdown in production by a third producer (Aventis Pasteur), as the company worked to remove the preservative thimerosal from its product. The remaining manufacturer, GlaxoSmithKline, was able to increase its supply temporarily, but a nationwide shortage still occurred (GAO, 2002).

Pricing

Pricing of DTaP has mirrored general industry pricing trends. From 1977 to 1982, the government price for DTP vaccine was quite low ($0.15 per dose in the public sector, $0.19 to $0.37 per dose in the private sector). By the mid-1980s, however, prices for many vaccines had climbed dramati-

BOX 2-2 Continued

cally. Between 1983 and 1986, for example, the cost of a single dose of DTP vaccine increased from $0.45 to $11.40 in the private sector and from $0.42 to $3.01 in the public sector (Sing and Willian, 1996). When Lederle's DTaP entered the market in the early 1990s, its prices were more than four times higher than those for the DTP product. The differences between CDC contract prices and private-sector prices have remained fairly constant; contract prices averaged 57.7 percent of private-sector prices between 1993 and 2002.

In 1997, CDC used DTaP contract negotiations to pilot a set of policies that represented a shift from a winner-take-all approach to multiple supplier contracts and allowed contractors to lower their prices during the contract period to compete for market share. After 2 years, these provisions were extended to all CDC vaccine contracts. As a result, manufacturers' contract prices began to converge, starting in 1997 and continuing through early 2001. In April 1998, all four manufacturers were selling at $7.00 per dose.

This stable pricing situation continued until the withdrawal of Baxter-North American and Wyeth in April 2001 and the temporary reduction in DTaP production by Aventis as it worked to remove thimerosal from its product. By January 2001, the nation was experiencing a recurrence of DTaP shortages. Prices have risen once again—to approximately $12.00 per dose.

The Future

DTaP is likely to become the platform on which larger combination vaccines will be built, combining five, six, seven, or more antigens into a single shot. In December 2002, the FDA licensed the first of the new combination DTaP-based vaccines. Developed by GlaxoSmithKline, the new vaccine combines five antigens: diphtheria, tetanus, and acellular pertussis (DTaP); hepatitis B (HBV); and polio (IPV) (Food and Drug Administration [FDA], 2002). Larger combination vaccines of this kind have already been introduced successfully in the European market. In addition, Glaxo-SmithKline has developed and licensed in other countries four other DTaP-based combination vaccines, including two that combine DTaP with Hib (*Haemophilus influenzae* type b) vaccine, a potential next candidate for the U.S. market (SmithKline Beecham, 2000).

As the nation faces both old and new challenges in reducing morbidity and mortality from communicable diseases, it is important to understand the complex nature of vaccine development and use, which sits at the intersection of four domains: science, public opinion, government policy, and private-sector market forces. Perhaps the key lesson learned from this brief history of DTaP is that all four domains will continue to evolve, sometimes in surprising ways.

SOURCE: Adapted from Fine (2003).

reducing barriers to entry for foreign producers—conflicts with desires to protect the quality of the vaccine supply and to assure safety for the diverse U.S. population.

Despite some recent interest in the development of government production or government-owned, contract-operated production (often referred to as "GoCo") of vaccines (IOM, 2001; NVAC, 2003), a broad consensus has emerged that only a thriving private vaccine industry has the production and R&D capacity to meet the nation's growing vaccine needs (IOM, 2000a). A diminished role for private industry could result in periodic shortages, total loss of supply of certain vaccines, price instability, and decreased investment in R&D.

THE SETTING OF NATIONAL VACCINE POLICY

The vaccine enterprise has experienced unprecedented turmoil and change in areas ranging from pricing and shortages to globalization and technological developments. Thus, the validity of key assumptions that have guided national vaccine policy to date is eroding. Vaccine policy has been essentially static, operating as if these changes have not occurred. New policies and strategies are necessary to guide the national immunization effort over the coming decades. How will this guidance emerge, and is the current planning apparatus up to the task?

Planning authority for vaccine policy resides in numerous agencies and independent bodies that have separate areas of responsibility. Conflicts can emerge among the objectives, plans, and regulatory decisions of these different entities. Looking to the future, questions of vaccine policy include which vaccines will be developed and produced, how safe and effective they will be, who should receive them, how much they are likely to be worth, how much they will cost, who should pay for them, and how they will be supplied to the public. Such questions are addressed in an uncoordinated fashion by multiple agencies with very different perspectives:

• *National Institute of Allergy and Infectious Diseases (NIAID)*. NIAID is the NIH institute responsible for establishing basic research funding priorities for immunization, which in turn influence the development of future vaccines. Private industry also plays an independent role in vaccine development, bringing vaccines from basic research to commercial development according to its assessment of which vaccines represent the most viable markets.

• *Food and Drug Administration (FDA)*. The FDA influences which vaccines come to market, the timing of releases of new vaccines, and the competitive structure of the industry. Moreover, through its impact on regulatory and production costs, the FDA indirectly influences prices and company returns on investment, which affect vaccine supplies and innovation. The FDA's broad regulatory influence hinges on two key policy levers—the standards it sets for efficacy and safety, and the manufacturing and administrative costs of compliance.

• *National Immunization Program (NIP)*. The NIP is the entity within CDC responsible for developing and implementing public health policy regarding vaccines. Its roles include negotiating federal vaccine contracts, providing grants and assistance to states, conducting immunization surveillance, studying vaccine safety, and coordinating public health programs nationally.

• *Advisory Committee for Immunization Practices (ACIP)*. ACIP is an advisory committee that determines which vaccines will be recommended for inclusion in the schedule of recommended vaccines. The schedule influences the accepted national standards of care for immunization. In addition, ACIP determines which vaccines will be included in the VFC entitlement. ACIP recommendations resulted in a virtual doubling of federal expenditures on vaccines (from $500 million to $1 billion) with the approval of the pneumococcal conjugate vaccine.

• *National Vaccine Program Office (NVPO)*. NVPO is an office within DHHS that conducts strategic planning for the NIP and provides liaison with the major immunization stakeholders, including other federal agencies, states and municipalities, providers, manufacturers, and consumers. While charged with performing a centralized planning and coordination role, NVPO has yet to demonstrate its ability to reconcile the competing interests both within and outside the government, perhaps because of inadequate resources.

• *National Vaccine Advisory Committee (NVAC)*. NVAC is an advisory committee to NVPO on matters of research, availability, safety and effectiveness, and public health associated with vaccines.

ACIP currently plays the pivotal role in this regulatory scheme, a role that bridges the supply side of the market (the industry and the FDA, which regulates it) and the demand side (the market for vaccines); the government programs that pay for vaccines; and CDC, which negotiates their prices and fosters public access (see Figure 2-1).

ACIP not only makes recommendations for the use of vaccines by children and adults but also determines whether a vaccine will be provided free to children through the VFC program. ACIP also has substantial influence on sources of payment since it controls billions of federal entitlement dollars. It is sometimes criticized for creating unfunded mandates to state and private insurers without sufficient consideration of the consequences for these stakeholders (France, 2000).

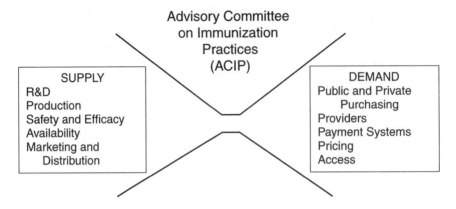

FIGURE 2-1 Central role of ACIP in vaccine policy.

The recommendation process begins with FDA approval for licensure of a new vaccine product. ACIP then begins considering whether and under what circumstances the vaccine should be recommended for use by the public. The American Academy of Pediatrics (AAP), through its Committee on Infectious Diseases (also known as the Redbook Committee), coordinates closely with ACIP in order to provide direction to the AAP professional membership that is consistent with ACIP's recommendations. The American Academy of Family Physicians (AAFP) also coordinates its recommendations with ACIP. The recommendations of both the AAP and the AAFP become standards across the medical community.

ACIP is a 15-member panel of experts appointed to 4-year terms by the DHHS Secretary (CDC, 2001a). Appointees must undergo a thorough conflict and bias review to determine their eligibility. ACIP includes scientific and medical experts in relevant fields of medicine and biology, as well as a consumer representative. The committee also has 19 nonvoting liaison members, who represent medical professional societies and other key groups, and 8 ex-officio members representing other federal agencies. Nonvoting members may participate in workgroup meetings, where a great deal of the actual work of ACIP is conducted. They may also be allowed to vote in specific cases designated by the ACIP executive secretary, such as when conflicts of interest exclude voting members. The committee is staffed by CDC; the executive secretary, who coordinates the committee, is a member of the CDC staff. ACIP holds three regular meetings each year, plus meetings of emergency consultation workgroups when necessary.

Issues considered by ACIP in making its recommendations include safety, efficacy, cost-effectiveness, feasibility, and risk–benefit ratios. Background work leading to the committee's recommendations is conducted by ad hoc workgroups, which can include voting and nonvoting members and CDC staff. Consultants and vaccine company representatives may provide data and technical assistance. The last step in the recommendation process is approval by the CDC director and publication in CDC's *Morbidity and Mortality Weekly Report*. ACIP reviews each recommendation at 5-year intervals to assess the need for changes. In addition to its full recommendations, ACIP can make permissive recommendations in the form of suggestions for the use of vaccines when the committee cannot clearly define the group at risk for the disease the vaccine is designed to prevent.

ACIP does more than simply make recommendations; it wields power beyond its mission, design, or authority. By default, it plays a pivotal role in vaccine policy by determining the market for vaccines, influencing prices, and setting a benchmark of sorts for the cost–benefit threshold for new vaccines. But this is a role for which ACIP may not be particularly well suited because it is not structured to perform such a broad public policy function. ACIP exhibits two principal limitations in this regard.

1. *Lack of authority beyond CDC*. ACIP is influential, but its statutory reach is limited. For example, its planning horizon for new vaccines is limited because it cannot anticipate the timing of FDA approvals. As soon as a vaccine has been approved by FDA, however, a 90-day clock starts ticking; and once it runs out, states are required to provide approved vaccines through Medicaid. In contrast, in the overall VFC program, vaccines need be provided only once a federal contract price has been negotiated. If ACIP is able to approve a new vaccine within this window and further approve its inclusion in VFC, CDC must still negotiate a contract before the vaccine will be covered by VFC. An expensive vaccine, such as pneumococcal conjugate, can create a burden for states, which must purchase the vaccine directly and must do so without benefit of the discounted federal contract price. State legislative action may also be required to secure additional funding for vaccines. If state funding is delayed, some private providers may need to purchase the vaccine at high prices and without assurance of compensation. In the case of pneumococcal conjugate vaccine, ACIP delayed publication of its recommendation until a price could be negotiated with the manufacturer; as a result, states and providers were financially responsible for vaccine purchases (Fairbrother and Haidery, 2002).

Private insurers may also face difficulties in paying for new vaccines not included in their annual budgets or premium calculations. They may choose to defer coverage until the next contract period or provide coverage at a loss. Provider groups that are globally capitated by health plans may face the same problem but with fewer resources to enable them to provide the vaccines at a loss (IOM, 2003a).

For vaccines included in the VFC program, only a few state Medicaid programs will reimburse private clinicians for the use of privately purchased vaccine that is available under the federal contract, even in the case of shortages when publicly purchased vaccine may not be available. However, most Medicaid programs will reimburse clinicians for needed vaccine for which no federal contract price exists (e.g., tetanus–diphtheria, adult pneumococcal, meningococcal), although others will not (Freed and Cowan, 2002).

To address these problems, AAP has recommended closer coordination of licensing, approval, and purchasing, with a target of 60 days after licensure for establishment of public and private price. AAP has also recommended that the federal government provide emergency funds with fixed annual appropriations to buy newly licensed vaccines for public programs in the interim between a recommendation by ACIP, AAP, and AAFP and incorporation of the expenditures in the regular budget cycle.

Once ACIP has issued a new vaccine recommendation and the federal contract for that vaccine has been negotiated, states must begin providing the vaccine through the VFC program. States may want to provide the newly recommended vaccine to non–VFC-eligible children for whom they provide other recommended vaccines. Doing so is becoming increasingly difficult, however, because of the high prices of recently recommended vaccines (Freed and Cowan, 2002).

The issuance of a new recommendation can be particularly problematic financially if the recommendation is released (and the federal contract negotiated) after federal and/or state funding decisions have already been made. Even when recommendations are anticipated before funding decisions have been made, these decisions are based on projections of need and uptake, which may not be accurate. Several states have noted, for example, that the annual federal funding decisions did not adequately account for the rapid uptake of pneumococcal conjugate by providers in the funding awards to states (Freed and Cowan, 2002).

2. *Need for appropriate economic decision-making expertise, data, and criteria.* Studies on the cost-effectiveness of vaccines imply that vaccines represent one of the best investments in public health. But vaccines are not inherently cost-beneficial; their cost-effectiveness depends on the price charged (Jacobs and Meyerhoff, 2001). In the existing system, ACIP has the responsibility for determining whether it is in the interests of the nation to utilize and pay for a vaccine, based on its cost and benefit to society. Cost-effectiveness is considered, but ACIP usually assesses the data without advance knowledge of the federal contract price or the costs of

production. In the case of pneumococcal conjugate vaccine, cost-effectiveness studies reviewed by ACIP underestimated the actual price. In the context of supply shortages, industry exit, and disincentives to innovate, ACIP's limited consideration of cost may represent an overly narrow perspective. Furthermore, the composition of the committee—infectious disease experts, physicians, and public health officials—may be ill suited to such economic analysis.

As a result, ACIP may be poorly equipped to deal with vaccines that are likely to emerge in the future. Vaccines are increasingly being introduced at higher prices. Also, there is a trend toward vaccines that target conditions other than contagious diseases and thus do not possess the traditional spillover effects characteristic of the majority of vaccines that prevent highly contagious diseases. Some new vaccines may have less-favorable cost–benefit profiles, and new combination vaccines may have costs and benefits not captured in traditional cost–benefit analysis. For example, Jacobs and Meyerhoff (2001) argue that the ACIP decision on pneumococcal conjugate vaccine did not meet conventional standards for cost-effectiveness. Regardless of whether this assessment is correct, it signals a major change in thinking about vaccines that will likely require new models of assessment and regulation.

FINDINGS

- Government is deeply involved in the immunization enterprise, a role that reflects the public-good and spillover characteristics of vaccines.
- Government policy toward vaccine R&D is inconsistent: it both promotes and discourages the development of new vaccines.
- While states continue to take principal responsibility for immunization infrastructure and delivery, it can no longer be assumed that they will share responsibility for vaccine purchase with the federal government.
- It cannot be assumed that private insurers will continue to share responsibility for covering immunizations.
- The assumption of a stable supply of vaccines produced by a healthy private sector can no longer be made.
- The current approaches to vaccine prioritization and immunization system planning are inadequate, as currently structured, to deal with the changing nature of vaccines and vaccine economics.

Public and Private Insurance Coverage
Summary of Findings

• An estimated 13.8 percent of children between birth and 5 years of age are underinsured (that is, have private insurance that does not include immunization benefits).

• Half of all adults aged 18–64 lack immunization coverage; 32 percent of this population (29 million adults) is considered to be at high risk.

• The proportion of children and adults without immunization coverage may increase as a result of current trends in insurance benefits and the increasing cost of the recommended vaccines on the immunization schedule.

• Insurance coverage and patient cost sharing are among the important factors influencing rates of immunization.

• The current vaccine financing system is fragmented and prone to funding delays; the result is missed opportunities and institutional barriers to immunization.

• Public vaccine financing programs have led to some crowd-out of private immunization coverage, and attempts to limit crowd-out have met with mixed success.

• Increasing vaccine costs, crowd-out of private-sector financing, and federal funding delays place significant stress on state financing mechanisms, prompting limits on state contributions to immunization programs.

3

Public and Private
Insurance Coverage

Immunization is financed through private health insurance, public safety net programs, and patient out-of-pocket spending. The source of coverage[1] varies substantially by age (see Table 3-1). Private insurance covers 52 percent of children aged 0 to 5 years for immunizations, and public programs cover about 34 percent. The remaining 14 percent of children are underinsured; as noted in Chapter 1, this population is defined here as those who have insurance that does not cover immunizations (see Figure 3-1). Children who have no insurance (public or private) are automatically covered by the Vaccines for Children (VFC) program; children who are underinsured can receive VFC-purchased vaccines only in federally qualified health centers and in their doctors' offices in some states that have expanded the VFC program with state dollars.

Americans aged 65 or older are almost universally covered for immunizations through Medicare. Adults aged 18–64 are covered less frequently for immunizations than either children or the elderly (see Figure 3-2). Private insurance covers about 41 percent of this population for immunizations, and public programs cover about 9 percent. The remaining 50 percent are either underinsured or uninsured. Unlike children, adults who are uninsured are not covered by any public programs until they become eligible for Medicare.

While older adults have Medicare coverage, adults under age 65 have virtually no safety net coverage for immunization. Only 17 percent of

---

[1]*Coverage* can refer to either the rate of immunization in a population or insurance enrollment. Throughout this report, the term is used exclusively to mean insurance enrollment.

TABLE 3-1 Insurance Coverage for Immunization by Age Group, 2000

Category	Number Covered (in thousands)	% of Population Category
U.S. Population	281,400	
Children 0–5		
Medicaid-enrolled	4,649	18.3
SCHIP—Medicaid expansion	241	0.9
SCHIP—Stand-alone	771	3.0
Native American—VFC-eligible	261	1.0
Private insured—immunization covered	13,143	51.8
Underinsured for immunization	3,494	13.8
Medicare-enrolled (disabled-ESRD[a])	194	0.8
Uninsured	2,619	10.3
Subtotal	25,372	100.0
Children 0–17		
Medicaid-enrolled	12,058	15.9
SCHIP—Medicaid expansion	690	0.9
SCHIP—Stand-alone	1,961	2.5
Native American—VFC-eligible	261	0.3
Private insured—immunization covered	42,113	54.6
Underinsured for immunization	11,195	14.5
Medicare-enrolled (disabled-ESRD[a])	517	0.7
Uninsured	8,406	10.9
Subtotal	77,201	100.0
Adolescents and Adults 18–64		
Medicaid-enrolled	10,582	6.0
Private insured—immunization covered	72,050	40.9
Underinsured for immunization—not high risk	38,270	21.7
Underinsured for immunization—high risk	20,680	11.7
Medicare-enrolled (disabled-ESRD[a])	4,778	2.7
Uninsured—not high risk	21,805	12.3
Uninsured—high risk	8,229	4.7
Subtotal	176,394	100.0
Adults Aged 65+		
Medicaid-enrolled	3,293	5.9
Private insured	20,761	30.6
Medicare-enrolled	31,733	57.0
Uninsured	245	0.4
Subtotal	56,032	100.0

[a]End-stage renal disease.
NOTE: Percentage totals may not add due to rounding.
SOURCES: Coverage data from U.S. Census Bureau, 2002; underinsurance data based on an analysis by Wood, 2003; calculations by the committee.

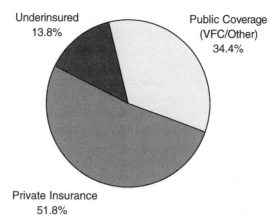

FIGURE 3-1 Insurance coverage of vaccination, children aged 0–5 (2000).
SOURCES: U.S. Census Bureau, 2002; calculations by the committee based on an
analysis by Wood (2003).

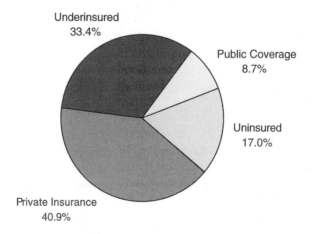

FIGURE 3-2 Insurance coverage of vaccination, adults aged 18–64 (2000).
SOURCES: U.S. Census Bureau, 2002; calculations by the committee based on an
analysis by Wood (2003).

adults aged 18–64 with chronic health conditions—and therefore at high risk for disease—had ever received the vaccine in 1999; only 31.9 percent of high-risk adults received an influenza vaccination (National Center for Health Statistics [NCHS], 2000).

State-funded county and city health departments are principally responsible for adult immunizations, and they are subject to capacity limitations and funding uncertainties. Fortunately, influenza immunizations are relatively inexpensive, and it has become common to administer them in shopping malls and employer settings. But these may not be appropriate settings for those who have chronic health conditions such as lung or heart disease or diabetes, especially those with limited mobility; and the paucity of coverage may limit the availability of these vaccines within the office-based practice setting.

The next two sections of the chapter provide a more detailed look at public and private coverage, respectively. The final section addresses the key barriers that currently constrain the ability of the immunization system to achieve the nation's immunization goals.

PUBLIC INSURANCE COVERAGE

Funding for both vaccine purchase and immunization infrastructure has historically been shared by the federal government and the states (see Chapter 2). While expenditures on vaccine purchase are increasingly determined by entitlement programs such as VFC and Medicaid, expenditures on infrastructure are largely discretionary and vary considerably from state to state. Table 3-2 summarizes the various sources for public funding of immunization.

TABLE 3-2 Public Immunization Funding, Fiscal Years 1999 and 2002 (in millions of dollars)

Funding Source	1999			2002		
	Federal	State	Total	Federal	State	Total
Section 317	448	NK	448	628	NK	628
VFC	467	NA	467	990	NA	990
Medicaid	70	57	127	90	69	159
Medicare	115	NA	115	255	NA	255
Total	1,100	57	1,157	1,963	69	2,032
% Change				78%	21%	76%

NOTE: N/A = not applicable; NK = not known.
SOURCES: FY 1999: IOM, 2000a; FY 2002: CDC, 2002e.

Public coverage for immunization includes both safety net programs designed to provide access for disadvantaged populations and non–safety net programs, such as health benefits for veterans, military personnel, and civilian government employees. These programs are described in depth in a recent IOM report (IOM, 2000a) and are briefly reviewed below.

Vaccines for Children

The Vaccines for Children (VFC) program was established by a 1993 amendment to the Social Security Act as an entitlement to provide federal funds for the purchase of vaccines for children under 18 years of age in four categories: Medicaid-eligible, uninsured, Native American/Alaska Native, and children who receive vaccines at federally qualified health centers (FQHCs). VFC funds are available to underinsured children only at FQHCs.

VFC works as follows. After recommending that a vaccine be added to the schedule of recommended vaccines, the Advisory Committee on Immunization Practices (ACIP) takes a separate vote for inclusion of the new vaccine in the VFC program. If the ACIP recommendation is approved by the administrator of CDC, the vaccine is automatically included in the VFC entitlement and must be provided free of charge to all eligible children. CDC then negotiates a discounted federal price with the manufacturer. CDC allocates to each state a credit balance based on the estimated number of recipients, which the state can use to order vaccine supplies from the manufacturer at the discounted federal price. States purchase vaccines and either stockpile them for distribution to registered providers or make arrangements with the manufacturer to deliver the vaccine directly to providers. By providing free vaccines to private providers for administration to VFC-eligible children in their medical homes, VFC has resulted in a large shift of public immunization from the public to the private delivery system (IOM, 2000a) (see Chapter 2). The creation of VFC also transferred a significant financial burden for vaccine purchase from the states to the federal government. States were no longer obligated to purchase childhood vaccines from their state-funded Medicaid budgets.

Section 317 Vaccines

Section 317 of the Public Health Service Act was established in 1963 to provide states with discretionary grants for vaccine purchase and infrastructure support through two types of funding: (1) direct assistance (DA) funds, which make up the majority of Section 317 funds received by immunization programs for vaccine purchase; and (2) financial assistance (FA) funds, which typically support program infrastructure but since 1999 have also included support for the purchase of vaccines for which there is no federal contract, such as tetanus and diphtheria vaccines and adult vaccines for hepatitis B, influenza, and pneumococcus.

Over the last decade, states have experienced a disruptive Section 317 funding cycle. Until the early 1990s, infrastructure had received minimal federal support. In response to the measles outbreak of 1989–1991, Section 317 funding for infrastructure development expanded dramatically. Because states were unable to ramp their programs up rapidly to utilize this funding, they experienced high levels of "carryover" funds. In response, Congress reduced infrastructure funding sharply in 1997, precisely at the time when many states were beginning to establish programs (Freed et al., 2000). States can use only minimal amounts of VFC funding for infrastructure; therefore, state health departments sought to replace the Section 317 cuts with new state revenue allocations, with generally limited success.[2] A previous IOM committee recommended an increase in federal funding of $75 million per year for infrastructure. This level was subsequently approved by Congress and included in the fiscal year 2001 and 2002 federal budgets.[3]

State and County Programs

States and counties provide safety net coverage for immunization through public clinics and a variety of targeted outreach programs. These programs are funded by a variety of sources—state general funds, federal maternal and child health block grants to the states, public health service block grants, federal programmatic grants, private foundations, and federal Section 317 grants.

Direct state funding to immunization programs for vaccine purchase is highly variable (Freed and Cowan, 2002). Several states provide no such funding. In many states that do have state funding for vaccine purchase, the funds are earmarked for adult vaccines or special programs (e.g., to support a new law requiring immunization for hepatitis B for entry to school). State legislatures typically appropriate general revenue funds for vaccine purchase, but financial support may also be provided through an ongoing mechanism to generate funds through a specific tax or surcharge or insurer contribution. State Medicaid and State Children's Health Insur-

---

[2]Twenty-one states provide direct infrastructure funding; only four states provide state funding that exceeds 40 percent of their infrastructure budgets (Freed and Cowan, 2002).

[3]The Department of Health and Human Services' fiscal year 2001 budget included a $42.5 million increase for fiscal year 2001, and the fiscal year 2002 appropriation included a $32 million increase (W. Orenstein, remarks to the IOM Committee on the Evaluation of Vaccine Purchase Financing in the United States, May 21, 2002).

ance Program (SCHIP) funds are also provided funds for vaccine purchase. Medicaid reimburses providers for the purchase of vaccines for those who are Medicaid-enrolled but not VFC-eligible (e.g., over 18 years of age). Vaccine purchases for children served under stand-alone SCHIP (i.e., non-Medicaid) programs must be made with state funds; 31 states have or are starting stand-alone SCHIP programs (Freed and Cowan, 2002).

States with universal purchase and enhanced-VFC programs expand eligibility for VFC vaccines by supplementing VFC vaccine purchases at federally discounted prices. They fund these efforts by providing a combination of Section 317 and state general revenue funds for the purchase of vaccines for non–VFC-eligible children. Enhanced-VFC states provide free vaccines to non–VFC-eligible and underinsured children who are seen in the public sector. In addition, state funds are used to purchase vaccines for underinsured children in the offices of private providers. There are currently 15 states with enhanced-VFC programs, while 14 states have universal purchase programs in which ACIP-recommended vaccines are made available to all children, regardless of insurance status (see Table 3-3). Universal purchase states tend to use a larger proportion of state funds relative to Section 317 funds for vaccine purchase. Some states exclude the most expensive vaccines (typically pneumococcal conjugate and varicella) from both enhanced-VFC and universal purchase programs (Freed and Cowan, 2002).

Medicare

Medicare covers virtually all Americans aged 65 and over—about 32 million in all—through Medicare Part B, as well as about 5,000 children and adults who are disabled or who have end-stage renal disease (Wood, 2003). Medicare coverage for immunization, however, is limited to influenza and pneumococcal vaccines, although others can be administered when shown to be medically necessary (i.e., not preventive in nature).

PRIVATE INSURANCE COVERAGE

The nature and scope of coverage for immunization tend to vary by the type of insurance plan. For example, health maintenance organizations (HMOs), which have traditionally emphasized preventive services, frequently provide immunization as a basic covered benefit. Preferred provider organizations (PPOs) and indemnity insurance, on the other hand, have more limited immunization benefits. The first four columns of Table 3-4 show coverage levels for different types of health plans according to recent surveys.

TABLE 3-3 State Vaccine Purchase Financing Systems

VFC Only	Enhanced VFC	Limited Universal Purchase	Universal Purchase
Alabama	Florida[a]	Connecticut[b]	Alaska
Arkansas	Georgia	Nevada[b]	Idaho
California	Illinois[c]	North Carolina[b]	Maine
Colorado	Kentucky[a]	North Dakota[b]	Massachusetts
Delaware	Maryland	South Dakota[b]	New Hampshire
District of Columbia	Michigan[a]	Vermont[b]	New Mexico
Hawaii	Minnesota		Rhode Island
Indiana	Montana[a,c,d]		Washington
Iowa	Nebraska[c,e]		
Louisiana	New York		
Mississippi	Oklahoma[a,c]		
Missouri	South Carolina		
Ohio	Texas[c]		
Oregon	Utah[a]		
Pennsylvania	Wyoming		
Tennessee			
Virginia			
West Virginia			
Wisconsin			

[a]Moved from a VFC-only to enhanced-VFC system in 1999.
[b]Moved from a universal purchase system to a limited universal purchase system in 1999.
[c]PCV-7 (and varicella in Illinois) available only for VFC-eligible children.
[d]In process of changing back to VFC-only system.
[e]Private providers can choose to receive some state-purchased vaccines for non–VFC-eligible children.
SOURCE: Freed and Cowan, 2002.

In addition, the relative market share of different types of insurance plans affects the rate of private immunization coverage. According to the most recent Kaiser Family Foundation-Health Education and Research Trust (KFF-HRET, 2002) survey of employers, the growth of private HMOs plateaued in 1996 at 31 percent of covered employees and had declined to 26 percent by 2002. Point-of-service plans, many of which are similar in benefit design to HMOs, plateaued in 1999 at 25 percent of covered employees and had declined to 18 percent by 2002. PPOs, on the other hand, grew steadily between 2000 and 2002, and now represent 52 percent of employer-based enrollment. The last three columns of Table 3-4 indicate enrollment trends for each type of insurance plan. Given the more limited range of immunization benefits within PPOs relative to HMOs and point-of-service plans, immunization rates are likely to decline should these trends continue, if only because of the change in the relative market share of insurance plan types.

TABLE 3-4 Insurance Coverage for Immunization and Employer-Based Market Share by Type of Insurance Plan

| Plan Type | Rate of Coverage | | | | Market Share | | |
| | Childhood | | | Adult | | | |
	1996	1998	2001[a]	2001[a]	2000	2001[a]	2002
Health maintenance organization	97%	99%	80%	66%	29%	37%	26%
Point-of-service plan	NA	98%	78%	58%	22%	20%	18%
Preferred provider organization	82%	86%	79%	57%	41%	50%	52%
Indemnity insurance	68%	79%	NA	NA	8%	NA	5%

[a]Based on data from the National Survey of Employer-Sponsored Health Plans 2001, conducted by Mercer Human Resource Consulting, Inc. Survey excluded indemnity option. SOURCES: Wood, 2003; KFF-HRET, 2002.

The rates of private insurance coverage indicated in Figures 3-1 and 3-2 somewhat overstate the level of private coverage as a source of payment for immunization because they omit patient cost sharing in the form of deductibles and copayments. These costs are difficult to estimate, but indications are that they represent a significant portion of immunization payments. For example, a recent National Immunization Survey found that 79 percent of privately insured children had some sort of payment associated with their last immunization visit (CDC, 2002f), although the median amount was only $9.96. In a study by Lieu et al. (1994b), 66 percent of privately insured immunization patients at public clinics stated that they were using the public clinic rather than another source because of cost.

Concerns have been raised about the potential drift toward reduced benefits on the part of all types of insurance plans. The committee has no specific evidence that insurance plans have dropped immunization coverage, but believes that immunization benefits are likely to follow trends in other benefits, especially as the total cost of vaccination rises relative to that of other benefits. In 2002, 17 percent of workers were in companies reporting a decline in benefits from the previous year (KFF-HRET, 2002). Between 2000 and 2002, deductibles for PPO in-plan coverage grew by 48 percent. Employer health premiums increased by 12.7 percent between 2001 and 2002, the second year of double-digit increases. There is concern that the higher expected prices of new vaccines and the increasing number of recommended vaccines will lead to a further erosion of immunization benefits and continuing increases in cost sharing (Robinson, 2002).

Patient cost sharing is increasingly used by employers as a way to shift some of the cost burden of health care to employees. But the economic rationale that has propelled cost sharing into wide use among insurers from the 1970s is its effect on patient demand. By placing some financial responsibility for the use of medical care on consumers, cost sharing encourages them to limit frivolous utilization and to shop for lower-priced services. The use of cost sharing in the case of immunization may indeed encourage price shopping (as is indicated by the high numbers of insured patients seeking immunizations at public clinics because of costs [Lieu et al., 1994b]). On the other hand, cost sharing may discourage some people from receiving immunizations at all. Thus, while there are desirable aspects of cost sharing, in the vaccine context it is potentially counterproductive in that it works directly against the policy of promoting the utilization of vaccines for the public good.

Defined contribution plans, although not yet a significant market presence, have the potential to grow rapidly (Gabel et al., 2002); indeed, 6 percent of firms report that they are "very likely" to adopt such a plan within the next 5 years (KFF-HRET, 2002). These plans allow consumers to allocate dollars from a medical savings account as they wish. The growth of these plans may have a negative effect on rates of immunization, as some consumers in these plans are likely to forego such preventive benefits.[4]

The ability of private insurers to drop coverage or increase cost sharing is constrained by federal and state insurance mandates. Federal maintenance-of-effort laws were intended to prevent crowding out of private coverage with the passage of VFC. Immunization benefit mandates have also been enacted in 28 states. In 18 of these states, immunization benefits are exempt from deductibles, and 12 states prohibit insurance plans from charging patients deductibles and copayments (American Academy of Pediatrics [AAP], 2003). State laws, however, apply only to state-regulated plans; self-funded employer health plans, which represent about half of enrollees in private insurance plans,[5] are exempt from state regulation under the Employee Retirement and Income Security Act (ERISA). Furthermore, interpretation and enforcement of state mandates vary widely (Swartz, 2003).

---

[4]Some plans fully fund preventive benefits to address this concern.

[5]In 2000, 48 percent of enrollees in private employer-sponsored health plans were in plans that were self-funded and therefore exempt from state insurance regulation under the federal Employee Retirement Income Security Act (Bureau of Labor Statistics, 2003).

In universal purchase states, health insurance plans usually provide coverage for vaccines but do not bear their costs because the state provides the vaccines free of charge to providers. These plans do, however, pay provider fees associated with vaccination. Several states have excluded certain expensive vaccines from their universal purchase programs because of severe budget constraints, and one state has returned to a nonuniversal program. If this should become a trend, it is not clear that private health insurers would be willing and/or able to quickly resume funding for immunizations.

Given the potential for increases in vaccine costs (as discussed in Chapter 1), no one can predict with certainty how insurers will address immunization benefits in the future. However, both health plans and employers have expressed alarm about the rate of increase in vaccine expenditures and the financial pressures that could ultimately lead to the further reduction or elimination of immunization benefits (Swartz, 2003).

There are two principal concerns regarding private coverage of immunization. First, erosion of coverage shifts the financial burden to both individuals and public payors. For some individuals, this may mean that they do not have access to immunization services. For states, this erosion adds to budgetary stresses, delays in funding, and increased fragmentation of financing (issues discussed below). Second, the difficulty of accurately measuring the shift from private insurance coverage to the public sector makes it difficult to estimate vaccine budget requirements to assure adequate funding.

BARRIERS TO A WELL-FUNCTIONING IMMUNIZATION FINANCE SYSTEM

As noted in Chapter 1, the combination of public and private insurance coverage and vaccine provider arrangements has resulted in successfully immunizing children in remarkably high numbers. Four key finance-related barriers, however, constrain the ability of the system to achieve the nation's immunization goals. These barriers—gaps in coverage and patient cost sharing, funding delays, fragmentation, and a crowding out of private insurance—are discussed below. Other barriers include socioeconomic status, education, public awareness, and administrative barriers (Santoli et al., 1998; Szilagyi and Rodewald, 1996). Such factors are also reviewed, followed by an assessment of the relative importance of finance-related and other barriers and a discussion of the important issue of pockets of need.

Gaps in Coverage and Patient Cost Sharing

While the existence of gaps in insurance coverage has been established, the effect of these gaps and of patient cost sharing on rates of immunization has yet to be demonstrated. Until recently, vaccines were relatively inexpensive and within the means of the poor. It is therefore reasonable to ask how much of a difference coverage and cost sharing really make in immunization rates today. If they have a significant effect, public policies to increase coverage or reduce out-of-pocket costs would clearly be warranted; otherwise they would not.

A handful of recent studies address these issues (see Table 3-5), but the evidence is not conclusive. The studies fall into five categories: provider-reported data on immunization by insurance status, patient- or parent-reported data on reasons for lack of immunization, comparison group studies between free-vaccine and non–free-vaccine states, before-and-after studies in states initiating free-vaccine programs, and randomized trials based on different cost-sharing levels. These studies are further grouped into either childhood or adult immunization.

Childhood Immunization

- Lurie et al. (1987) examined data from the RAND Health Insurance Experiment (HIE) and found that children and adults in plans with free preventive care (including vaccines) had 20 percent and 70 percent higher rates of immunization, respectively, than those in plans with copayment. The usefulness of this study for present purposes, however, is limited by the fact that the key dependent variable—the degree of cost sharing—applies not just to immunization, but also to other types of care received during the same visit. Thus the costs associated with a provider visit may be important, but this is not necessarily the case for the costs associated with the immunization itself.

- Rodewald et al. (1997) evaluated a statewide program in New York that enabled children to receive free vaccines from providers throughout the state. Controlling for age, he found that the program increased immunization rates by 30 percent for those with no previous insurance and by 32 percent for those with Medicaid coverage. (The study took place before the VFC program was introduced.)

- In an interview study conducted by Nace et al. (1999) in Tennessee, 19 percent of physicians cited inadequate insurance as the principal reason for the lack of immunization among patients. A lack of insurance was cited by 16 percent of parents; 11 percent specifically cited underinsurance.

- Taylor et al. (1997) evaluated private physicians among a geographically dispersed sample of participants in the American Academy of Pediatrics (AAP) Pediatric Research in Office Setting network. Using a regression that controlled for education, size of metropolitan area, and child's age, he found no significant differences in immunization attributable to free vaccines. However, the practices evaluated, by virtue of self-selection into the AAP research network, may not be representative of practices across the United States.

• Freed et al. (1999) conducted a survey to determine the impact of universal purchase in North Carolina and found that immunization had increased in all insurance categories. The largest increases were in the Medicaid (4.1–6.3 percent) and uninsured (8.6–9.2 percent) categories. The underinsured experienced increases of 4.1–6.3 percent. Freed, however, did not control for other variables that might have affected immunization rates over this period.

• Recent data from CDC's National Immunization Survey suggest that, at least for expensive vaccines such as varicella, there is a substantial (12 percentage point) differential in immunization rates between insured and underinsured children (CDC, 2002g). This analysis, however, did not control for confounding variables, such as income and education, and therefore may be misleading.

Adult Immunization

• Using data from the 1998 National Health Interview Study, Pleis and Gentleman (2002) showed that high-risk adults aged 18 to 64 were twice as likely to get immunized for influenza if they had insurance. The regression analysis controlled for age, sex, race, poverty status, health status, region, and smoking.

• A well-designed study by Ohmit et al. (1995) found that a free-vaccine intervention strongly increased rates of immunization for influenza relative to controls in three of four test groups, after controlling for age, gender, smoking, and high health-risk conditions. Unfortunately, the study included multiple interventions and did not distinguish the incremental impact of free vaccines from the effect of intensive outreach efforts.

• Randomized trials conducted by Ives et al. (1994) in Pennsylvania and Satterthwaite (1997) in New Zealand found extremely high impacts of free vaccines: rates of immunization were 18–28 percent higher than in the control group in the former study and 66 percent higher in the latter. However, because both studies included multiple interventions, the incremental effects of free vaccines cannot be isolated.

• Nexoe et al. (1997) conducted a randomized controlled trial among 13 general practices in Denmark. It was found that free vaccines increased

TABLE 3-5 Studies of the Impact of Insurance and Cost Sharing on Immunization Rates

Author	Findings	Study Period	Design	Sample Size
Children				
Lurie (1987)	Enrollees in plans with free preventive care had between 20% and 70% higher rates of immunization than those in copayment plans, according to age: • Ages 0–6: 20% • Ages 17–34: 36% • Ages 35–65: 70%	1974–1982	Randomized trial in Ohio, Washington, Massachusetts; assignment to insurance plans with varying coverage. Cost sharing not specific to vaccines.	3,823
Rodewald (1997)	Up-to-date immunization rate for diphtheria–tetanus–whole-cell pertussis (DTP)/oral polio vaccine (OPV)/measles–mumps–rubella (MMR) increased as a result of enrollment in the program. Increases varied by previous coverage: • No previous coverage: 30.4% • Full previous coverage: no significant difference • Medicaid enrollment: 32.2%	1991–1993	Comparison of immunization status before and after enrollment in an in upstate New York program providing free vaccines to children up to 222% of poverty level. Tried to control only for age.	1,835
Nace (1999)	Inadequate insurance cited by 19% of physicians as reason for incomplete immunization by 2 years of age. "Insurance does not cover immunizations" reported by 11% of parents; 16% if "no insurance" included.	1997	Survey of parents of 2,400 children under age 3 in Tennessee.	110 physicians, 1,180 parents

Taylor (1997)	No significant difference between children enrolled in the copayment plan and the free-vaccine plan.	Early 1990s	Comparison group survey of pediatricians in 11 states; two samples. Not necessarily representative of private practices.	857,772
Freed et al. (1999)	Percentage of children up to date at ages 12 and 24 months higher for post–universal purchase cohort than for pre–universal purchase cohort. • 12 months: Increases ranged from 1.3 percentage points (privately insured) to 9.2 percentage points (uninsured and Medicaid). • 24 months: Increases ranged from .5 percentage points (privately insured) to 8.9 percentage points (Medicaid).	1994–1995	Before–after random survey of parents in North Carolina. Confounding factors not controlled for.	2,767
CDC (2002f)	Varicella immunization rate for insured children is 80.4% and for underinsured children is 68.1%. No statistical difference for the 4:3:1:3 series.	2001	Preliminary data from CDC National Immunization Survey Insurance Module. National survey with provider verification of immunization status. Confounding factors such as income and education not controlled for.	2,811

continued

TABLE 3-5 Continued

Author	Findings	Study Period	Design	Sample Size
Adults				
Ives et al. (1994)	Intervention, including free vaccines and outreach, increased flu immunization rates by 18–28% over rates in the control group.	1989–1991	Randomized trial of elderly in five Pennsylvania counties. Controlled for sex, marital status, and high-risk medical conditions. Results confounded by multiple interventions.	1,989
Nexoe et al. (1997)	Among patients 65 and older, 72% offered free vaccines were immunized, vs. 49% who paid the usual fee.	1995	Randomized trial among patients of general practices in Denmark. Out-of-pocket immunization cost ($40–60) higher than is typical in the United States.	13 providers, 585 patients
Pleis and Gentleman (2002)	High-risk adults aged 18–64 with insurance had a rate of influenza immunization double that of those without insurance (16% vs. 32%). Adults aged 65 or older with insurance had triple the rate of influenza immunization of those without insurance (66% vs. 23%).	1995, 1998	CDC's National Health Interview Survey. Regression analysis controlling for age, sex, race, poverty status, health status, region, and smoking.	17,317, 32,440

| Ohmit et al. (1995) | Statistically significant increase in influenza immunization rate occurred in the intervention group (free vaccines, provider fees, and outreach) relative to the control group. | 1989–1992 | 2,978 | Comparison group study in clinics and offices in southwest Michigan. Regression model controlled for age, sex, health status, and smoking. Results confounded by multiple interventions. |
| Satterthwaite (1997) | Immunization rates increased by 66% for those offered free immunization vs. those charged $20. | Not reported | 1,860 | Randomized trial among elderly (>85) clients of general practices in New Zealand. Results confounded by multiple interventions. |

immunization rates by 47 percent, but the cost of immunization for the control group was excessively high at US$40–60.

Many of the above studies have shortcomings with respect to the questions relevant to research on vaccine finance. For example, the impact of underinsurance, a key focus of this report, is addressed only indirectly in most of these studies, which therefore rely upon the impact of provider out-of-pocket costs or indirect evidence. The literature also does not examine directly the question of why insurance and cost sharing matter, given the relatively low price of most vaccines. However, research on private physicians' referral of patients to the public sector for immunization, which is discussed in the next chapter, may offer more insight. This literature suggests that the relationship between immunization and insurance/cost sharing may have less to do with demand than with physicians' decisions to provide vaccines to broad classes of patients on the basis of their insurance coverage and physician-perceived ability to pay. Finally, few of these studies control for confounding factors, such as nonfinancial barriers (e.g., access to providers), discussed later in this chapter, that may affect immunization rates.

While these studies are unsatisfying in many respects, taken together they suggest that insurance and cost factors do influence immunization rates. This is the case especially for lower-income children without other insurance and for adults who lack compulsory immunization through state school entry requirements.

Funding Delays

Bottlenecks in the current immunization system can result in delays in coverage for vaccines. One such bottleneck results in delays between Food and Drug Administration (FDA) approval, addition to the recommended schedule, and negotiation of a contract between CDC and the manufacturer. Such delays create hardships for budget-strapped states and health plans. A second bottleneck often occurs with federal and state discretionary appropriations that are required to fund vaccines for non–VFC-eligible children and adults. The result can be a two-tier system in which providers can immunize VFC children but must turn away children who do not qualify for VFC or bear the costs themselves. These bottlenecks can discourage providers from immunizing children and can impede adult immunization efforts as states shift Section 317 and state funds away from adult programs to address urgent childhood vaccine shortfalls.

Fragmentation

The complex immunization financing system results in fragmentation of coverage and several associated problems. Multiple funding sources make it difficult for providers to determine the eligibility of patients. This is particularly true for underinsured patients. If private providers are uncertain whether a patient is covered, they are more likely to refer that patient to a public clinic. Even public clinics must worry about eligibility. For example, VFC vaccines can be used for underinsured children, but only in FQHCs.

Moreover, many patients are likely to shift in and out of eligibility with significant frequency (IOM, 2000a, 2002d). Households that depend on seasonal employment or are cut from Medicaid rolls during periods of fiscal austerity are examples of the turnover that can occur in safety net programs. As an example, 40 percent of children in California lose Medicaid coverage each year (IOM, 2000a). This situation creates financial risk for providers, who may not receive payment if eligibility is determined incorrectly. As noted above, providers may choose to refer patients rather than deal with the complexity of the system, thereby creating fragmentation of care for the patient, additional burdens for the patient or parent, and possibly delayed or missed immunizations. Providers are also placed in the awkward position of providing immunizations for some but not others on the basis of insurance coverage.

Another form of fragmentation relates to fees paid to providers for administering vaccines. Under VFC, vaccine purchases and administration fees have two separate funding sources. The federal government provides an entitlement for vaccine purchases, while administration fees are reimbursed through state-supported Medicaid payments. Depending on the status of federal negotiations and state appropriations, providers may receive vaccine reimbursement but no administration fee, fee but no vaccine reimbursement, and other possible combinations. Furthermore, provider administration fees vary widely across states. In many states, provider payments barely cover vaccine costs, resulting in increases in referrals to the public sector (Fairbrother and Haidery, 2002). This situation in turn makes it more difficult to estimate state discretionary funding needs.

Crowd-Out of Private Insurance

Historically, attempts to address gaps in the immunization system have led to a crowd-out of private-sector insurance (AHSRHP, 2001; see also Chapter 2). Crowd-out occurs when public programs displace private markets. For example, public housing partially displaces private rentals and ownership when individuals who would otherwise have rented or purchased in the private market obtain free or subsidized housing. Similarly, public financing of immunization can result in private providers referring patients to public immunization clinics (as discussed above) and insurance companies dropping immunization benefits. Because the public safety net system is there to immunize those without access to private providers, many of these individuals will receive appropriate immunizations at the right times. But many gaps exist in the public safety net coverage for immunization. Also, referrals from private providers increase the chances of missed opportunities, leading to longer periods of vulnerability to vaccine-preventable diseases.

Other Barriers

While the above analysis argues for the importance of finance-related barriers to the achievement of national immunization goals, noneconomic factors are also significant (see *Calling the Shots* [IOM, 2000a] for detailed discussion of these factors). Evidence for the importance of noneconomic factors includes the observation that populations with high socioeconomic status sometimes have low immunization rates, (IOM, 2000a; Orenstein et al., 1999). For example, a study of privately insured children of parents working in a large corporation revealed that only 65 percent of the children were up to date with the 4:3:1 series at age 2 (Fielding et al., 1994). Noneconomic factors that influence immunization rates include both personal and systemic variables (Bates and Wolinsky, 1998).

Personal Variables

Personal characteristics, including socioeconomic status and educational attainment, have been linked to immunization rates. In a small multivariate analysis of children, the majority of whom lacked private health insurance, Bates and Wolinsky (1998) found that underimmunization at age 2 was associated with mothers who were unmarried, had multiple children, did not reside with a grandparent, did not receive adequate prenatal care, and lived in poverty. Other studies have demonstrated positive relationships among parents' education level, family income, and immunization rates (Ortega et al., 2000; Hughart et al., 1999). On the other hand, when other socioeconomic variables are controlled for, race is not usually an important factor (Bates and Wolinsky, 1998; Marks et al., 1979).

Patient beliefs are also important correlates of immunization rates. One study found that more than 75 percent of parents had delayed bringing a child in for immunization at some time because of the child's minor illness, even though the vaccination was not contraindicated (Abbotts and Osborn, 1993). Bates and Wolinsky (1998) found a significant positive association between immunization at age 2 and perceived "control and responsibility over life events" and an unexpected negative association with the perception of the benefits of immunization.

Others have looked at the impact of incentives for immunization, such as giving toys, money, or discount coupons. However, there is little evidence indicating the effectiveness of such techniques (IOM, 2000a).

System Variables

A wide range of variables relating to the immunization delivery system has been assessed, including the immunization site, vaccine availability, and provider variables.

As noted earlier, the provision of vaccinations in the medical home is a hallmark of the VFC program. The implementation of VFC, as well as similar state-level universal purchase programs, coincided with substantial increases in immunization rates, suggesting that the medical home may make an important difference in the rates achieved (Freed et al., 1999; Nace et al., 1999). Research findings are mixed, however, on the contribution of a routine source of care to these increases. Data from the 1988 National Health Interview Survey (NHIS) indicated that before VFC was enacted, 90 percent of children already had a routine source of care, although only 77 percent had been fully immunized by age 2 (St. Peter et al., 1992). These results were affirmed by the 1993 NHIS, which revealed that 90 percent of children who were not up to date had a medical home (Tatande et al., 1996). Likewise, a recent study found no significant association between immunization rates and immunization within the medical home (Ortega et al., 2000). On the other hand, Bates and Wolinsky (1998) found that children are more likely to be up to date at age 2 if they have a medical home and if their provider is a private physician.

States have also promoted immunizations at medical sites not traditionally used for the purpose, such as hospitals, pharmacies, and nursing homes (Briss et al., 2000; IOM, 2000a). Some have promoted nonmedical sites for immunization, such as Women, Infants, and Children (WIC) program sites, schools, child care centers, stores, malls, and patients' homes. The effectiveness of these interventions has not been established through research, however. One concern regarding such strategies is that the appropriate medical record for immunization may not be present at the point of service. States have also attempted to improve access at existing sites by extending hours, adding staff, and providing express services at immunization clinics.

Provider-level variables affect immunization rates as well. Clinicians defer immunizing patients with surprising regularity because of a child's illness, a large number of shots being administered during a single visit, or parental concerns. As noted above, they may also refer patients to public clinics because immunization is not financially rewarding; high rates of such provider referrals, even among insured patients, are well documented (Zimmerman et al., 1997) (see Chapter 4 for a full discussion of this issue). In addition, immunization involves many clinical and administrative tasks, including purchasing vaccines, managing inventories, determining immunization status and eligibility, counseling parents, administering vaccines, recording and reporting immunization, and conducting reminders/recalls. Almost all of these tasks have expanded in recent years as a result of the growing number of vaccines and the complexity of the schedule, the rising cost of vaccines, and the recent shortages of both childhood and adult vaccines. Many providers consider the financial rewards for immunization in the form of current fees to be inadequate (AAP, 2001a).

Clinicians may also lack sufficient vaccine supplies at the time of service. They may voluntarily elect to limit supplies because of the increasing cost of purchasing vaccines and the uncertainty of reimbursement (Freed et al., 2002a), or they may be unable to purchase adequate supplies because of supply disruptions. While there is no direct evidence of reduced immunization rates or increased disease incidence as a result of recent vaccine shortages, there is some indirect evidence that a supply disruption may adversely affect provider immunization practices (Oram et al., 2001). For example, CDC has reported that 52 percent of states suspended school immunization requirements as a result of the tetanus vaccine shortage (Orenstein, 2002c).

Providers may also lack efficient systems for vaccine administration, such as reminder/recall systems, assessment and feedback processes, standing orders (which allow nonphysicians to administer vaccines without direct physician supervision), and even simple checklists (Briss et al., 2000; IOM, 2000a). Evidence supporting the benefits of such systems is limited, however, and their adoption by providers has not been widespread (Darden et al., 1999; IOM, 2000a).

Unavailability of a child's complete immunization record to the clinician is a critical factor in underimmunization (Stokely et al., 2001). This situation often occurs when families move within or across states or switch providers, and it is exacerbated by the increasing complexity of the immunization schedule and the fragmentation within the immunization financing system discussed above. There is growing evidence that the use of electronic vaccine registries can significantly improve the accuracy of immunization records (Boyd et al., 2002; Davidson et al., 2003; Stille and Christison-Lagay, 2000); the impact of such registries on immunization rates, however, has not been clearly demonstrated. An alternative strategy is to have patients or parents retain "handheld" immunization records; here too, however, there is little evidence that this approach is effective, and it may in fact cause administrative problems (Dickey and Petitti, 1992; IOM, 2000a).

The increasing availability of combination vaccines may improve immunization rates. The current vaccine schedule requires as many as five injections during a single visit. Two or more of these are often deferred because of parental concern about the fear and pain involved in multiple injections (Glode, 2001). There is a clear parental preference for combination vaccines. A survey by Meyerhoff et al. (2001) found that it is worth a median of $8.00 to parents to avoid having their child receive an additional injection. Another study found that reducing the number of shots from four to three is worth a median of $25, from three to two is worth $25, and from two to one is worth $50 (Lieu et al., 2000b). Also, reducing the required number of injections can significantly reduce administrative time (Pellissier et al., 2000). There is, however, no direct evidence on the impact of combination vaccines on immunization rates. There are also potential drawbacks, including the presence of competing combinations with various overlapping antigen menus and subtle immunologic differences that may create confusion and/or administrative burden for busy practitioners (Le, 2001).

Mandatory immunization, such as that required for school entry, appears to be effective in increasing immunization rates. All states adopted such school laws during the 1970s and 1980s (IOM, 2000a), and immunization rates increased dramatically. But the relative impact of school entry laws compared with other factors has not been determined. Also, the impact of school entry requirements occurs well after most vaccinations are typically administered: 20 of the 23 recommended childhood vaccinations are normally completed by 18 months of age. The increasing use of day care requirements addresses this shortcoming, but such requirements have not been as widely implemented as those for school entry. Other mandates are now being widely applied for nursing homes. There is however, insufficient evidence of the effectiveness of any of these requirements (IOM, 2000a).

Relative Importance of Finance-Related and Other Barriers

Several studies directly compare the importance of finance-related and other factors. One study found that cost was the most important reason given by parents for having their children immunized at a public health clinic. Of those interviewed, 63 percent had come to the public clinic because of its lower cost, and 79 percent of families interviewed rated this as an important factor in choosing a public health facility (Lieu et al., 1994b). Other factors cited include convenient location, no appointment needed, recent relocation, and other access advantages. In another study, lack of insurance coverage was deemed the third most important reason for incomplete immunization by age 2 (cited by 16 percent of parents), after waiting time (33 percent) and child ill at the time of appointment (21 percent) (Nace et al., 1999).

Developing a full understanding of the relative importance in immunization of the finance-related and personal and systemic variables discussed above will require substantial additional research. No clear evidence has emerged that can be used to rank the relative importance of these factors. It is clear, however, that both sets of factors are important and require attention if full immunization is to be achieved. If finance-related barriers—the primary focus of this report—are not addressed, strategies that address noneconomic barriers will not be fully effective.

Pockets of Need

Uninsured children fare well under the current system: they are categorically covered under VFC and can receive free vaccines in their medical home or from any VFC provider or clinic. Ironically, the biggest coverage gap for children is among those who have private insurance coverage—21 percent of insured children aged 0–5 lack coverage for vaccines (Wood, 2003). VFC statutorily excludes these children because they are "insured." Fourteen states address this gap by providing state-funded coverage for the underinsured. In these states, children can receive free vaccines through their own provider, regardless of their insurance coverage. But parents of children in the other 36 states must either pay out of pocket or take their children to a public health clinic to obtain free vaccine.

The same problem is experienced by children who are enrolled in stand-alone SCHIP programs. While Medicaid-eligible children are categorically qualified to receive free VFC vaccines, children in stand-alone SCHIP states, such as California, are technically "insured," and the Centers for Medicare and Medicaid Services (CMS) has ruled that they are excluded from VFC coverage. These children still receive vaccines from their SCHIP provider, but without VFC funding.

Estimating the Number of Underinsured

Estimates of the number of underinsured children vary considerably and are not deemed highly reliable. CDC is considering ways to improve estimates of underinsurance. The committee considered several estimates, which were summarized earlier in Table 3-4.

A recent Partnership for Prevention study used by Wood (2003) estimates that 21 percent of privately insured children aged 0–5 have private insurance that excludes immunization. This suggests that 3.5 million children aged 0–5 are underinsured—13.8 percent of this age group. Wood points out that some of these underinsured are covered through state universal purchase programs in 14 states. On the other hand, this estimate excludes the children who are covered by insurance for immunizations but face prohibitive copayments and deductibles.

Preliminary first-quarter results from the 2002 National Immunization Survey indicate that 7.3 percent of children (aged 0–17) have some kind of insurance (either public or private) that excludes immunization (CDC, 2002d). Meyer and Waldman (2002), using data from KPMG and Health Research and Educational Trust (HRET) surveys, estimates that about 8 percent of children are underinsured for immunizations. The IOM (2000a) study cited earlier also uses KPMG data to derive an estimate of 5 percent for the underinsured population aged 0–17.

Studies examining the insurance status of individuals using public clinics support the above estimates of the incidence of underinsurance. Lieu et al. (1994b) found that about 16 percent of immunization patients at public clinics were underinsured. A more recent analysis of data from the 2002 National Immunization Survey found that 44–63 percent of children vaccinated in public health clinics in South Carolina and California were underinsured (CDC, 2002i).

Immunization Insurance Benefits for Adults

The coverage picture for adults is far less positive than that for children. Like children, adults face the problem of underinsurance. According to the Partnership for Prevention survey cited above, 59 million adults aged 18–64 have private insurance that does not include immunization benefits (Wood, 2003). In addition, more than 30 million adults under age 65 are uninsured. Unlike uninsured children, who are categorically covered by VFC, uninsured adults have no safety net immunization program. Thus, a total of 89 million adults under 65—50 percent of this age group—lack coverage for immunizations.

Older persons generally require fewer routine vaccinations than children; but adults at high risk for vaccine-preventable diseases may need to be immunized against pneumonia, influenza, meningitis, and hepatitis. (Table 3-6 shows the population at high risk for severe influenza or pneumococcal disease within various age groups.) More than 65,000 deaths from influenza and pneumonia occur annually, most among older adults (CDC, 2002b).[6] In contrast, about 300 deaths occur each year as a result of

---

[6]Note, however that the majority of these deaths are among those aged 65 and older. Some portion of these deaths are likely due to family decisions not to immunize because of extreme age or frail health.

TABLE 3-6 Adults Considered to Be at High Risk for Influenza or Pneumococcal Disease

Age group	Population	Percent of Age Group at High Risk	Population at High Risk	Population at High Risk and Uninsured	Population at High Risk and Under-insured	Annual Number of High Risk in Need of Publicly Purchased Vaccine
18–49	136 million	11%	15 million	2.7 million	5.0 million	7.7 million
50–64	43 million	100%[a]	43 million	5.5 million	16.0 million	21.5 million
Total adults 18–64	180 million	32%	58 million	8.2 million	21.0 million	29.2 million

[a]1995 recommendation is for 100% of this group to receive influenza annually and pneumococcal vaccine one time.
SOURCE: Adapted from Wood, 2003.

all vaccine-preventable diseases among children. In addition, 48,000 pneumonia and influenza hospitalizations occur annually among adults over age 65 (CDC, 2001a). The monetary burden of adult vaccine-preventable diseases is estimated to be greater than $10 billion per year (CDC, 2002c).

Although Medicare plans provide coverage for older adults for pneumococcal immunization (since 1981) and for influenza immunization (since 1993), immunization levels among older adults remain low. In 1997, 66 percent of this population received an influenza immunization, and a cumulative 50 percent had received a pneumococcal immunization—still well below the national goal of 90 percent established for each in *Healthy People 2010* (U.S. Department of Health and Human Services, 2000). Fortunately, many adults have access to influenza immunization sponsored by employers, retail stores, and shopping malls. This may partly explain the significant gain in immunization rates among this population in the last several years.

ACIP recommends pneumococcal vaccination for all adults over age 50, adults between age 18 and 64 at high risk—e.g., those with chronic diseases affecting the lungs, heart, immune system, and selected other organ systems—and all adults aged 65 and older (CDC, 2003f). Annual influenza vaccination is recommended for high-risk adults (aged 18–49) and for all adults over age 50. According to Wood, 58 million Americans, or 32 percent of adults under age 65, are considered to be at high risk for vaccine-preventable diseases (Wood, 2003). Half of these, about 29 million adults, have no coverage for immunizations.

FINDINGS

- An estimated 13.8 percent of children between birth and 5 years of age are underinsured (that is, have private insurance that does not include immunization benefits).
- Half of all adults aged 18–64 lack immunization coverage; 32 percent of this population (29 million adults) is considered to be at high risk.
- The proportion of children and adults without immunization coverage may increase as a result of current trends in insurance benefits and the increasing cost of the recommended vaccines on the immunization schedule.
- Insurance coverage and patient cost sharing are among the important factors influencing rates of immunization.
- The current vaccine financing system is fragmented and prone to funding delays; the result is missed opportunities, institutional barriers to immunization.
- Public vaccine financing programs have led to some crowd-out of private immunization coverage, and attempts to limit crowd-out have met with mixed success.
- Increasing vaccine costs, crowd-out of private-sector financing, and federal funding lags place significant stress on state financing mechanisms, prompting limits on state contributions to immunization programs.

Delivery Systems
Summary of Findings

- Private office-based providers administer the majority of publicly funded immunizations.
- The administrative burden associated with immunizing children is increasing.
- Provider reimbursement does not adequately reflect the increasing burden of immunization and creates uncertainty about payment.
- Variations and delays in both public and private insurance coverage for vaccinations create uncertainty about provider payment.
- Private providers refer patients to the public sector in large numbers in response to inadequate reimbursement and excessive administrative burdens.
- Public clinics may provide insufficient access and capacity to maintain a reliable safety net for children and adults who are uninsured for immunization or referred from the private sector for other reasons.

4

Delivery Systems

Adult and childhood immunizations are delivered through fairly distinct systems. This chapter begins by describing those systems and then reviews the specific tasks involved in providing immunizations and the mechanisms for provider reimbursement. The final section addresses barriers to achieving a well-functioning immunization delivery system.

DELIVERY OF ADULT AND CHILDHOOD VACCINES

Privately insured adult patients receive immunizations through private providers or frequently, in the case of influenza vaccine, at work or other non-medical sites. As noted earlier, however, the immunization safety net for adults is far more limited than that for children. In some states, counties bear the principal responsibility for adult immunization in the public sector (Freed and Cowan, 2002). Local health departments purchase influenza vaccine with local or county funds. In some areas, such as Los Angeles and Houston, local health departments receive state funding for adult vaccination.

Vaccines commonly provided to adults include viral influenza, hepatitis A and B, pneumococcal polysaccharide, and the 23-valent meningococcal vaccine. Many states also provide a significant amount of tetanus vaccine to the adult population. As the U.S. population ages, many states are expecting increased demand for influenza and meningococcal vaccines. Moreover, any changes in the recommendations of the Advisory Committee on Immunization Practices (ACIP) for viral influenza vaccine will have a significant impact on adult immunization budgets.

Some states are experiencing a significant increase in the use of hepatitis A and B vaccines with new programs targeting specific at-risk populations. Other states with large numbers of migrants also believe they will see an increase in demand for adult immunization services. In addition, the recent downturn in the economy will likely result in fewer adults having health insurance; and as a consequence, larger numbers will seek care (including immunizations) at public clinics (Freed and Cowan, 2002).

Childhood immunizations are provided to the public through two main venues: private office-based providers and public health clinics. Before the implementation of the Vaccines for Children (VFC) program, private providers generally immunized privately insured individuals, and public clinics immunized safety net populations. As discussed earlier, one of the goals of the VFC program was to increase the proportion of children who receive vaccines in their medical home. Almost overnight, VFC expanded the number of publicly certified immunization providers from about 3,000 public immunization sites to more than 40,000 public and private provider sites (IOM, 2000a; see also Chapter 2).

Over the past several years, the proportion of children receiving publicly purchased vaccine in the offices of private physicians has increased markedly. The shift in delivery of childhood vaccines from the public to the private sector has been documented extensively. For example, between 1994 and 1998, the National Immunization Survey reported a decrease from 24 to 17 percent in the proportion of families who received all immunization from public clinics (Fairbrother and Haidery, 2002). In some states, the shift was even more pronounced. In Washington State, for example, the public sector accounted for 80 percent of vaccine delivery and the private sector for 20 percent in 1994; by 1999 these figures had reversed. Before VFC, the public sector delivered 70 percent of the state's immunizations; but by 1999 that number had dropped to just 35 percent (Fairbrother et al., 2000). Other states, such as Minnesota and Pennsylvania, also reported reduced doses delivered in the public sector (Zimmerman et al., 2001), while some states, such as Maine and New Jersey, reported that virtually all their immunizations—90 percent—took place in the private sector (Fairbrother et al., 2000). Not surprisingly given these trends, physicians (Zimmerman et al., 1997) and nurse practitioners (Zimmerman et al., 2000) participating in national surveys revealed that they were referring fewer children to public clinics and were vaccinating more in their own offices. Table 4-1 provides estimates from state immunization programs of the proportion of publicly purchased vaccines administered in the private sector. While both public clinics and private providers have proven to be effective at providing immunizations to the public, both are currently under stress.

Public clinics remain an important safety net for those without access

TABLE 4-1 Proportion of Publicly Purchased Vaccines Administered in the Private Sector

≤60%	60–70%	70–80%	80–90%	>90%
Alaska	Alabama	Colorado	California	Connecticut
Arkansas	Florida	Georgia	Delaware	Hawaii
District of	Idaho	New Mexico	Massachusetts	Maryland
Columbia	Indiana	North Carolina	Minnesota	New Hampshire
Illinois	Iowa	South Carolina	Oregon	New York[a]
Kentucky	Michigan	Utah	Rhode Island	Pennsylvania
Louisiana	Mississippi	Wyoming	Virginia	Vermont
Montana	North Dakota			Washington
Nevada	Ohio			
Oklahoma	South Dakota			
Tennessee	West Virginia			
Texas				
Wisconsin				

[a]Does not include New York City.
NOTE: Based on estimates provided by state immunization program officials. Estimates not available for Maine and Nebraska.
SOURCE: Freed and Cowan, 2002.

to immunizations through the private sector. But the capacity of the public sector is finite, and its ability to absorb spillover from the private sector is limited. Community health centers, including federally qualified health centers (FQHCs),[1] are fiscally stressed; and their capacity to serve their client base—including their capacity to provide immunizations—has been threatened in recent years (IOM, 2002d). A recent report of the National Association of County and City Health Officials (NACCHO, 2003) notes that just under 75 percent of city and county health agencies provide direct immunization services.

Furthermore, underinsured patients can receive VFC vaccines only in FQHCs. As of 2001, there were 1,200 FQHCs operating 3,000 delivery sites, serving 10 million people each year (GAO, 2001). But in some states, access to these centers is limited. For example, Oklahoma has only 5 FQHCs operating 18 sites throughout the state.

Public delivery systems already struggle to address the flow of referrals from the private delivery system. Should the private provider ar-

---

[1]The term *community health center* (CHC) refers to nonprofit health clinics that provide primary medical care to underserved populations. They include both health centers that do and do not receive Section 330 grants from the Bureau of Primary Health Care. In 1992, an alternative term—*federally qualified health center* (FQHC)—was established. This term refers to CHCs eligible to receive Medicare payment (IOM, 2002d).

rangements that support the safety net immunization function break down, it may not be possible for public clinics to compensate. Tensions between the two systems are emerging. For example, Michigan officials, responding to increased referrals from private providers experiencing vaccine shortages, directed local health departments to cease providing immunizations to underinsured children (Wendland-Bowyer and Askari, 2002). While the public delivery system may be far from the breaking point, it is clearly under stress; and even gradual erosion of the system could lead to gaps in immunization.

Alternative approaches for administering vaccines may be useful in increasing immunization rates. The issue of using alternative settings is addressed in a recent IOM report (IOM, 2000a), which highlights the enormous expansion of access as a result of the VFC program and the resulting shift in immunization settings from public clinics to private providers. The evidence on the impact of this shift on immunization rates (reviewed in Chapter 3) is inconclusive. With neither a strong evidence base to suggest an alternative delivery structure nor a specific charge to address these issues, however, this committee did not consider alternatives to the current delivery system for immunizations.

THE WORK OF IMMUNIZING

The immunization of children and adults involves a number of clinical and administrative tasks.[2] Almost all of these tasks have expanded significantly in recent years as a result of the increasing number of vaccines and the complexity of the recommended schedule, the increasing cost of vaccines,[3] and the recent shortages of both childhood and adult vaccines. A review of the various tasks associated with providing immunizations is presented below.

Purchasing Vaccines

While many clinicians receive vaccines at no cost through the VFC-program, most clinicians (in non-universal purchase states) purchase additional stocks for both private and public patients who do not qualify for

---

[2]A more detailed list of tasks associated with providing immunization is contained in the report of a recent IOM workshop (IOM, 2003a).

[3]Other incidental costs have increased as well. A recent ruling by the Occupational Safety and Health Administration that "safe sharps" (retractable needles) be used for the administration of childhood vaccines rather than the current nonretractable needles will add an estimated $14 million annually to the administrative costs associated with immunization (AAP, 2001b).

VFC. As a result of the increased cost and growing number of vaccines in recent years (see Chapter 1), these purchases have become a sizable investment, typically tens of thousands of dollars for a busy pediatric practice. Providers frequently must price shop by contacting multiple vaccine distributors. Recent shortages have increased the complexity of this task.

For providers in capitation arrangements, expensive new vaccines and expanded eligibility have resulted in a significant cost burden on providers until new contracts can be negotiated. In California, this situation led to litigation (IOM, 2003a).

Delays in public funding and managed care contracts for new vaccines have also caused significant problems in physicians' offices (Freed et al., 2002a; see also Chapter 3). These problems have been especially acute in recent years as the cost of the recommended vaccine schedule has risen to the nearly $600 per child at undiscounted prices that most physicians must pay (CDC, 2003d,e). The introduction into the schedule of pneumococcal conjugate vaccine at $58 per dose (or $232 for the recommended four-dose series) adds to the total cost, exacerbating an already difficult situation. Pediatricians often provide a vaccine as soon as it is recommended by ACIP and the American Academy of Pediatrics (AAP), even though details of funding have not been worked out (Davis et al., 2002). This approach has worked with the introduction of the less-expensive vaccines of the past because many payors were reimbursed for the vaccines after the fact, and pediatricians were able to absorb the residual costs. With expensive new vaccines and substantial delays in public funding (as in the case of pneumococcal conjugate vaccine), however, pediatricians have had difficulty absorbing these costs.

The AAP has received reports from pediatricians who owe significant amounts of money for pneumococcal conjugate vaccines that they purchased anticipating eventual third-party reimbursement (Fairbrother and Haidery, 2002). Many found that the reimbursement they received did not adequately cover the price of the vaccine or that third-party payors were not providing reimbursement at all. The AAP has also received reports from physicians who had to take out lines of credit to meet payroll costs and remain open because of the loss of income they experienced in providing this vaccine. And the AAP has learned of physicians who, because of cost considerations, are contemplating referring children to a public clinic rather than providing the vaccine in the children's medical home.

Beyond problems of paying for vaccine, pediatricians are faced with an interim period during which some children are covered for the vaccine but not others, and the physician must either provide differential service depending on children's insurance status or find a way to pay for those children not covered. The problems this situation engenders go beyond those associated with bookkeeping.

Managing Inventories

In states without universal purchase programs, private providers who participate in VFC must maintain two separate stocks of vaccines for their patients—one for children eligible for state-purchased vaccines and one for those patients for whom they purchase vaccines in the private marketplace. Shortages or budgetary delays may deplete the public or private stocks of vaccine. Many states do not reimburse providers who use their stock of privately purchased vaccine for a child eligible for a state or federal government vaccine program. However, at least 14 states do allow trading of vaccine stock to replenish any privately purchased vaccine used in place of publicly purchased vaccine (or vice versa). Regulation and documentation of vaccine tracking range from highly structured to very informal.

Determining Immunization Status

Fragmented delivery and provider referrals make determination of immunization status difficult, even in states with registries (see also Chapter 3). This is because safety net patients may move seasonally or relocate frequently, may go to different providers for regular care and for immunization, and are unlikely to maintain good records of their immunization status. This situation, which is exacerbated by the increasing complexity of the immunization schedule itself, results in both under- and overimmunization (Feikema et al., 2000).

Determining Eligibility

Given the many different forms of coverage for vaccines, providers must determine which payor will cover an immunization. If a patient has private insurance, it may or may not cover immunizations. For patients without private coverage, the provider must determine eligibility for public programs, such as Medicaid, the State Children's Health Insurance Program (SCHIP), VFC, Medicare, or other state public assistance programs. Complicating this task is the frequent movement of patients in and out of eligibility. It may be impossible to determine private underinsurance status in advance without contacting the insurer. Furthermore, an insurer may provide coverage for immunization but exclude certain vaccines.

Counseling

Counseling parents has become considerably more difficult in light of an organized and vocal vaccine "backlash" that has created heightened concern about the safety of childhood vaccines. Many adults also have concerns about the safety of influenza vaccination (CDC, 1999b).

Administering Vaccines

The additional work involved in administering a vaccine during a routine patient visit has been documented through time and motion studies (Fontanesi et al., 2001; LeBaron et al., 1999). LeBaron found, for example, that administration of vaccines incurs an additional 3.5 minutes of clinical time, which results in an estimated 32.3 million person-hours required to immunize a cohort of children born during a 1-year period with the 4:3:3:1 schedule.

Recording and Reporting Immunization

There has been an increase in requirements for reporting immunizations to health plans, employers, state registries, and indicators used by regulatory/accreditation bodies (e.g., the National Committee for Quality Assurance's [NCQA] Health Plan Employer Data and Information Set [HEDIS]). Rask et al. (2000) estimates that the costs of reporting to immunization registries alone range from $0.24 per immunization if fully automated to $3.24 in a manual system. The annual cost for a provider to participate in a registry can be nearly $25,000. On the other hand, studies have also shown that participating in registries can result in substantial efficiencies for clinicians. A study by All Kids Count showed that average costs to retrieve, use, update, and refile medical records are, on average, three times higher than those for participating in a registry (National Vaccine Advisory Committee [NVAC], 1999). Registries can streamline immunizations for clinicians by simplifying reminder/recall campaigns, eliminating vaccine wastage due to duplicate immunizations, and standardizing reports and school certificates (Horne et al., 2000).

Issuing Reminders and Recalls

Recent vaccine shortages have resulted in many patients being turned away. It has then become necessary to undertake expensive recall efforts once vaccine supplies have been replenished.

PROVIDER REIMBURSEMENT

As noted earlier, providers are reimbursed for both vaccines and administration fees. This reimbursement occurs in several ways (see Table 4-2):

• VFC vaccines are received free, and administration fees are paid for by the state Medicaid program.
• For vaccines purchased for public-sector patients who do not qualify for VFC (e.g., Medicaid recipients aged 18–21), providers receive vaccine reimbursement and an administrative fee from the program that provides coverage (e.g., Medicaid or SCHIP). Provider fees for uninsured individuals are paid through state public health funds, possibly supported by Section 317 or federal block grant funding.

TABLE 4-2 Provider Payment for Vaccines and Administration Fees

Insurance Status	Vaccine Reimbursement	Paid By	Administrative Fees	Cost Sharing?
VFC-eligible	Free	VFC	National average = $7.10 2nd+ shots= $6.85	Permitted to charge copayment or balance bill, up to a given amount
Medicare	Based on Medicare fee-for-service cost index	Centers for Medicare and Medicaid Services (CMS)	Relative value unit (RVU) rate is $7.72 (average)	Permitted to charge copayment; no balance billing
Other public	If VFC, vaccine is free; otherwise, price set by state based on average wholsesale price (AWP)	State health department	State discretion, based on AWP or Medicare RVU	Depends on state
Privately insured	Set by each plan	Private health plan	Set by each plan	Yes—limited by state laws

SOURCE: Personal communication, A. Shefer, CDC, July 12, 2002.

- Under Medicare, preventive immunizations are limited to adult influenza, pneumococcal vaccines, and hepatitis B and are covered by Medicare Part B.
- Private insurance either reimburses the vaccine cost plus the administration fee or includes these costs in a capitation amount that is paid to the provider.

None of these mechanisms guarantees that the amount reimbursed for the purchase of a vaccine will cover its actual cost. Vaccine reimbursements are usually based on a statewide or national average price benchmark, such as the average wholesale price. Providers hope that the vaccine reimbursement and administration fee, combined, will at least cover the price of the vaccine (Glazner et al., 2001). In certain cases, private providers can bill patients (both private and public) for some percentage of the difference between their usual charge and the amount reimbursed.

Provider administration fees for immunization vary widely from state to state. Each state determines its fees based on Current Procedural Terminology (CPT) codes 90471 and 90472 for the first and each subsequent vaccine administration, respectively. According to the 2001 Medicaid Reimbursement Survey, state fees range from $2.00 to $13.33 for CPT 90471 and $1.15 to $13.33 for CPT 90472 and average $7.10 and $6.85, respectively (AAP, 2002). SCHIP fees are either included in a capitation rate or reimbursed in a manner similar to that for Medicaid.

Medicare administration fees to providers are used as a benchmark for Medicaid and private insurers in setting fees. CMS fees are based on three measures of the resources that go into the service (measured in terms of relative value units [RVUs])—physician work, practice costs, and malpractice. Because adult vaccination occurs within the context of other medical activity, CMS concludes that it entails no incremental "work" over and above the office visit, and therefore sets the physician work component to zero. The result is a calculated fee of $7.72.

The American College of Physicians–American Society of Internal Medicine (ACP–ASIM) conducted a survey as part of their Adult Immunization Initiative and found that 85 percent of general internal medicine physicians believe reimbursement for immunization is inadequate and is a barrier to their practice's ability to provide immunization services (American College of Physicians–American Society of Internal Medicine [ACP–ASIM], 2002). Moreover, the AAP and other organizations recently asked CMS to consider the higher burden on physicians imposed by pediatric to adult immunization. CMS responded by doubling the fee from $3.98 per vaccine in 2002 (AAP, 2001a; ACP-ASIM, 2001; American Academy of Family Physicians, 2001). In addition, 63 percent of all private and public payors, including Medicaid, have adopted components of the Medicare Resource-Based Relative Value Scale (RBRVS) to determine fees.

New combination vaccines, such as GlaxoSmithKline's new diphtheria–tetanus–acellular pertussis (DTaP)–inactivated poliovirus (IPV)–hepatitis B vaccine, may result in lower administrative costs. However, they will also likely be more expensive to purchase. The net effect will not be known until experience with new combinations can be evaluated.

Several studies have demonstrated that financial incentives, including administration fees, play a role in immunization rates (Fairbrother et al., 1999; Szilagyi et al., 2000a,b; Wood and Halfon, 1996; Zimmerman et al., 2000, 2001). Cohen and Cunningham (1995) found a strong positive relationship between fees and preventive care measures. Other studies have looked at the connection between fees and referrals. New York State reformed its immunization system in 1994 by requiring first-dollar (i.e., no copayment) coverage of immunization and substantially increasing vaccine administration fees for providers. The proportion of private physicians who reported that they referred some or all children to public clinics for immunization decreased from 51 percent in 1993 to 18 percent in 1997 (Szilagyi et al., 2000a). This shift was reflected in coverage rates: in the inner city of New York in private offices seeing the poorest children, immunization rates for diphtheria–tetanus–whole-cell pertussis (DTP), polio, and measles–mumps–rubella (MMR) rose from 18 to 42 percent (Fairbrother et al., 1997).

BARRIERS TO A WELL-FUNCTIONING IMMUNIZATION DELIVERY SYSTEM

Three principal barriers to a well-functioning immunization delivery system can be identified: excessive provider burden, inadequate and uncertain provider reimbursement, and high rates of referral to public clinics among private physicians. Each of these barriers is reviewed below.

Excessive Provider Burden

The burdens associated with providing vaccines to both public and private patients are substantial and growing. Some of these burdens, such as the addition of vaccines to the schedule and the increased costs of vaccines, are unavoidable; but some burdens are due to systematic problems that could be addressed. These include the difficulty of determining eligibility and the risk to providers of doing so incorrectly, problems in determining immunization status, and the need to segregate vaccine inventories by payor.

Inadequate and Uncertain Provider Reimbursement

Current provider reimbursement does not reflect the increasing burden of immunization. Provider reimbursements for vaccine and administration fees often barely cover the costs of vaccine purchase. In many cases, providers lose money on immunization (Glazner et al., 2001). When confronted with inadequate compensation, providers may choose to immunize anyway and absorb the losses; or they may refer patients to public clinics (see below) (Fairbrother et al., 1996; Santoli et al., 1998; Szilagyi and Rodewald, 1996). While it is not clear how high provider fees should be, the evidence suggests that in the long run, inadequate compensation may compromise the viability of the private provider system for immunization.

In some cases, providers also face uncertainty about receiving payment for vaccines. This occurs, for example, when providers directly purchase vaccines for VFC patients because of delays in the federal contract, when shortages deplete stockpiles of VFC vaccines, or when reimbursement rates are not clearly established in advance (Freed et al., 2002a).

High Rates of Referral to Public Clinics

That physicians refer substantial numbers of children to public clinics is well documented, even when the children are eligible for free VFC vaccines (Lieu et al., 1994b; Zimmerman et al., 1997). The referral of large numbers of patients—even those who have private health insurance benefits for immunizations—from private providers to public health clinics indicates problems with the public–private system. Before VFC, many providers routinely referred patients to public clinics for immunizations rather than risk uncertain payment. After VFC, referrals declined dramatically as free vaccines became available to immunize a large proportion of the non-private patient population. However, while referrals were reduced by VFC, they were not eliminated. For example, Zimmerman et al. (1997) found that provider referrals within a practice varied according to insurance coverage (see Table 4-3). In 1995, 44 percent of physicians receiving free VFC vaccines remained likely to refer an uninsured child to a clinic. More surprising, 8 percent would even refer a child with insurance that covered vaccines. Lieu et al. (1994b) surveyed parents using public clinics for immunization. Her study revealed that, although 24 percent of those seeking immunizations at public clinics had private insurance and 34 percent had Medicaid, most in this group named cost as the main barrier to immunizations by office-based primary care providers.

Among providers' reasons for referring patients with privately insured immunization benefits to public health clinics are difficulty in de-

TABLE 4-3 Studies on the Impact of Insurance on Referrals

Author	Findings	Study Period	Design	Sample Size
Freed et al. (1999)	The proportion of children receiving immunizations from private providers increased from 63% for the 1994 cohort to 68% for the 1995 cohort.	1996	Pre- and post-VFC study (although pre-phase occurred during VFC implementation) with parents of children born in 1994 and 1995, with medical chart abstraction.	2,767
Lieu et al. (1994b)	Among those interviewed, 63% came to public clinic because of cost.	1992	Survey of patients at three public immunization clinics in California.	494
Rodewald et al. (1997)	For children aged 0–5, immunizations at public clinics declined 37% after enrollment; immunization by private providers increased 15%. For children aged 1–5, changes were 67% and 27%, respectively.	1992–1994	Survey of parents of children less than 6 years old recently enrolled in New York State insurance program covering immunization.	1,835
Ruch-Ross et al. (1994)	Percent likely to refer to public clinic: • Uninsured: 86% • Medicaid: 61% • Insured: 57% Percent of providers who referred some patients: • Free vaccine state: 27.8% • Not free vaccine state: 71.6%	1992	National survey of pediatricians (AAP members), controlling for physician age and gender, practice model, urban/rural, and universal purchase/non–universal purchase state.	1,246
Schulte et al. (1991)	Referrals by pediatricians increased 193% and by family physicians 391% between 1979 and 1988.	1979, 1988	Survey of pediatricians and family physicians in Dallas County.	381

		Year	Description	N
	Proportion of children referred increased 693%.			
	Inability of patients to pay cited by 70.4% as reason for referral.			
Szilagyi et al. (2000a)	In 1993, 51% referred; in 1997, 18% referred. Increases reportedly due to insurance mandate (61%) and VFC (60%). In 1997, physicians with no access to VFC vaccines were more than twice as likely to refer than those with such access (29% vs. 13%).	1993	Longitudinal survey of pediatricians and family physicians in New York State before and after state insurance mandate and VFC.	328
Zimmerman et al. (1997)	Percent likely to refer to public clinic: • Uninsured and unable to pay: 66% • Underinsured: 36% • Medicaid: 26% • Insured: 8% Among physicians receiving free vaccine, 44% likely to refer uninsured child; among those likely to refer. Cost as factor hindering timely vaccinations cited 5% (median).	1995	National survey of family physicians, pediatricians, and general practitioners.	1,236
Zimmerman et al. (1999)	Children are less likely to receive the first dose of the measles-mumps-rubella (MMR) vaccine on time from a provider who is likely to refer (69%) than from one who is unlikely to refer (81%).	1995–1996	Interviews with physicians and reviews of clinical records.	29

continued

TABLE 4-3 Continued

Author	Findings	Study Period	Design	Sample Size
Zimmerman et al. (2000)	Percent likely to refer to public clinic, if no access to free vaccines: • Uninsured: 67% • Medicaid: 27% • Insured: 7% Percent likely to refer to a public clinic if access to free vaccines: • Uninsured: 47% • Medicaid: 10%	1997	National survey of pediatric nurse practitioners.	252
Zimmerman et al. (2001)	Mean likelihood of referral decreased by 1.9 (on a scale of 0 to 10).	1990–1993, 1999	Longitudinal pre- and post-VFC survey of pediatricians, family physicians, and general practitioners in Minnesota and Pennsylvania.	281

termining eligibility, high costs of stocking vaccine inventories, and low payment rates for administering vaccines (as discussed above). It is apparent that the ability or willingness of a patient to pay for a vaccine may be less important than a provider's interest in supplying it, although both may be related to insurance status. Providers may, for example, choose to stock insufficient supplies and then marshal their limited supplies for their fully insured patients.

Referrals to public clinics can result in missed or delayed immunizations (Luman et al., 2002) and thereby seriously affect overall immunization rates (Fairbrother et al., 1996; Santoli et al., 1998; Szilagyi and Rodewald, 1996). Referrals can also result in fragmentation of care that increases the burden on parents, reduces continuity of care by introducing multiple providers, and distributes patient immunization records across multiple settings.

FINDINGS

- Private office-based providers administer the majority of publicly funded immunizations.
- The administrative burden associated with immunizing children is increasing.
- Provider reimbursement does not adequately reflect the increasing burden of immunization and creates uncertainty about payment.
- Variations and delays in both public and private insurance coverage for vaccinations creates uncertainty about provider payment.
- Private providers refer patients to the public sector in large numbers in response to inadequate reimbursement and excessive administrative burdens.
- Public clinics may provide insufficient access and capacity to maintain a reliable safety net for children and adults who are uninsured for immunization or referred from the private sector for other reasons.

Vaccine Supply
Summary of Findings

- The U.S. vaccine market is small relative to total expenditures on personal health services and pharmaceuticals. The entire global market for vaccines is roughly equivalent to the sales of certain individual blockbuster drugs.
- The supply of U.S. vaccines is becoming highly concentrated, resulting in limited backup capacity in the event of supply disruptions.
- Inadequate build-up of vaccine stockpiles has limited their remedial effect on recent shortages. The development of 6-month stockpiles would help to avert short-term disruptions in supply but would not address more fundamental concerns, such as the continuing loss of suppliers from the industry.
- The risks and costs to manufacturers associated with vaccine production have increased. Key factors include regulation, removal of the preservative thimerosal, and an increase in vaccine injury lawsuits.
- Food and Drug Administration (FDA) resources for vaccine regulation have not kept pace with the growth and complexity of vaccine products. FDA regulation has shifted from a focus on science to a focus on enforcement. This shift may increase the risks and costs associated with vaccine production without increasing safety.
- The pace of vaccine research and development (R&D), particularly in the discovery stage, is currently high, but commercial development is impeded by pricing and industry returns. Investment in production capacity for existing vaccines is especially problematic.
- FDA licensure requirements—including the increasing size of clinical trials, the requirement that companies build full production capacity before licensure, and the inadmissibility of clinical data from outside the United States for U.S. licensure—create substantial barriers to entry.
- The requirement for building full plant capacity in advance of approval may limit fixed capacity and increase the chances of shortages.
- Vaccine company investments in R&D on new vaccines have been shown to be sensitive to prices and expected returns on investment. Ensuring socially desirable levels of R&D may necessitate prices that are substantially higher than current prices for most routine childhood vaccines.
- By using its bargaining power to achieve substantial discounts in federal contracts, CDC may substantially undervalue vaccines and reduce industry incentives for investment in both R&D and short-run production capacity.

5

Vaccine Supply

Vaccines have eradicated smallpox and polio and prevented deadly and disabling diseases in thousands of Americans. Given their historically low cost and important benefits, vaccines represent one of the outstanding bargains in health care. Nonetheless, the vaccine supply today is surprisingly fragile. Just how fragile it is was brought to national attention by severe vaccine shortages in 2001 and 2002, which affected 8 of the 11 routine childhood vaccines. Such shortages have the potential to result in serious outbreaks of disease and can erode public health programs and infrastructure that have taken years to build. But the greatest threat is that the discovery and development of future vaccines, many of which are now well within reach, will be delayed or abandoned.

This chapter reviews the vaccine market in the United States and the context within which it functions. Discussed in turn are the size and growth of the vaccine market, vaccine production and the associated cost structure, research and development, concentration in the vaccine industry, regulation of the industry, pricing, vaccine shortages, the stockpiling of vaccines, and CDC contracting. The chapter ends by describing the key barriers to a well-functioning vaccine supply system.

SIZE AND GROWTH OF THE VACCINE MARKET

Vaccines are a very small enterprise relative to the pharmaceutical industry overall: vaccine revenues constitute only about 1.5 percent of global pharmaceutical sales (Batson, 2001). Global sales of all vaccines combined are roughly equivalent to the individual sales of such familiar pharmaceutical products such as Lipitor, Prilosec, and Zocor (Marketletter, 2002). In just three decades, the number of firms supplying routine vaccines to the United States dwindled to 5 companies that today produce all of the routinely recommended childhood and adult vaccines.

U.S. vaccine sales are estimated to be about $1.5 billion per year, one-quarter of the global vaccine market (about $6 billion per year) (Mercer Management Consulting, 2002). Most of the vaccines sold in the U.S. market are produced by four large pharmaceutical companies: Aventis Pasteur, GlaxoSmithKline, Merck, and Wyeth. Two of these companies—Merck and Wyeth—are U.S.-based; the others are based in Europe. A fifth, smaller company based in the U.K., Powderject, supplies adult influenza vaccine to the U.S. Vaccines represent a small fraction of the business of the four large companies and increasingly must compete with the companies' pharmaceutical divisions for internal resources (Arnould and DeBrock, 2002).

Mercer Management Consulting (2002) estimates that the global market for vaccines (childhood and adult) has grown approximately 10 percent per year since 1992. Globally, a significant proportion of the growth during the decade of the 1990s was the result of the worldwide effort to eradicate polio. The remainder of the market grew at an annual rate of only about 1 percent (Mercer Management Consulting, 2002). In the United States, 72 percent of the growth in revenues in the early 1990s resulted from the introduction of new vaccine products and 10 percent from the increase in the measles–mumps–rubella (MMR) dosage (from one to two doses) from 1990 to 1995 (Mercer Management Consulting, 1995). More recently, the introduction of childhood pneumococcal vaccine in 2000 nearly doubled the U.S. vaccine market.

Pediatric vaccines constitute the majority of the vaccine market (about 70 percent). Traditional childhood vaccines, such as MMR, polio, and diphtheria–tetanus–acellular pertussis (DTaP)—which represent the core of the U.S. national immunization system—are viewed by the vaccine industry as low-margin commodities. Projections of strong vaccine industry growth, however, spurred by new developments in recombinant technologies and other advances, have stimulated renewed interest in vaccines. Much of this interest is directed toward new therapeutic and cancer vaccines and adult vaccines for targeted risk groups. Some have suggested the possibility of a $10 billion market by 2010 (Hirschler, 2002). But the ability to bring new vaccines to market still involves extraordinary technical and regulatory challenges. Maintaining producer interest and stable sources of supply of routine childhood vaccines remains a significant challenge (Arnould and DeBrock, 2002).

Large, multinational producers sell vaccines through a two-tiered pricing system. Prices in developed countries are high—current prices in western Europe and the United States are comparable—while a large volume of vaccines is sold to the developing world at significantly lower, essentially marginal-cost prices. High-income countries generate about 82 percent of vaccine revenues but represent only 12 percent of doses (Batson, 2001). This system serves the needs of both the multinational companies and the developing countries. The large volume of global sales permits the vaccine companies to exploit economies of scale in production while earning high returns on sales to developed countries. European multinationals typically produce hundreds of millions of doses, while American companies produce tens of millions of doses (Mercer Management Consulting, 1995). This disparity in volume has resulted in higher average production costs in the United States than in Europe. (See also the later section on cost structure.)

VACCINE PRODUCTION

A large number of vaccines are licensed in the United States by domestic firms and foreign suppliers, taking into account multiple combinations, as well as vaccines that are not routinely used (see Tables 5-1 and 5-2). Some manufacturers are more active than others. For example, Wyeth has 16 licenses for vaccines in the United States and Merck has 13, while seven manufacturers have only 1.

While many pharmaceuticals are manufactured with relatively standardized chemical engineering processes, vaccine manufacturing is less standardized and less predictable. It often involves the complex transformation of live biologic organisms into pure, active, safe, and stable immunization components. Highly sterile, temperature-controlled environments are needed at each manufacturing step, and many vaccines must be maintained within a narrow temperature range during storage and delivery—referred to as the *cold chain*. Vaccines approved by the Food and Drug Administration (FDA) are subject to high standards of safety and quality assurance, including rigorous and pervasive review procedures in which each individual batch of vaccine is licensed—a procedure not required for pharmaceuticals (Hay and Zammit, 2002).

In addition, once in production, each batch must be tested and approved prior to release. Vaccines require both a product license application (PLA) and an establishment license application (ELA), while new pharmaceutical products ("new chemical entities" or NCEs) require only the former. The ELA certifies that the facilities, equipment, and personnel involved in the manufacturing process meet FDA standards and Current Good Manufacturing Practices. Furthermore, to obtain a facility license for a vaccine, a company must first create full production capacity for that vaccine (see the discussion below) (Hay and Zammit, 2002).

TABLE 5-1 Domestic Producers of Vaccines for the U.S. Market

Company	Generic Name	U.S. Approval Date
Bioport Corporation (Michigan Department of Public Health)	anthrax vaccine adsorbed	1970
Wyeth (Wyeth Laboratories, Inc.)	cholera vaccine	1952
Bioport Corporation	diphtheria and tetanus toxoids and pertussis vaccine adsorbed	1998
Bioport Corporation	diphtheria and tetanus toxoids adsorbed	1970
Bioport Corporation	diphtheria toxoid adsorbed	1998
Wyeth (Lederle-Praxis)	haemophilus b conjugate vaccine	1988
Merck & Co. (Merck, Sharpe, and Dohme)	haemophilus b conjugate vaccine	1989
Merck & Co.	haemophilus b conjugate vaccine and hepatitis B (recombinant) vaccine	1996
Wyeth (Praxis Biologics)	haemophilus B vaccine	1990
Wyeth (American Cyanamid)	haemophilus vaccine	1985
Merck & Co.	hepatitis B vaccine	1982
Merck & Co.	hepatitis-A vaccine, inactivated	1996
Biogen	hepatitis-B vaccine	1989
Wyeth (Wyeth Laboratories)	influenza virus vaccine	1945
Wyeth (Wyeth Laboratories)	influenza virus vaccine	1961
King Pharmaceuticals (Parkedale Pharmaceuticals)	influenza virus vaccine	1998
Merck & Co.	measles and mumps virus vaccine live	1973
Merck & Co.	measles and rubella virus vaccine live	1971
Merck & Co.	measles virus vaccine live	1963
Merck & Co.	measles, mumps, and rubella virus vaccine live	1971
Merck & Co.	mumps virus vaccine live	1967
Bioport Corporation	pertussis vaccine adsorbed	1998
Greer Laboratories	plague vaccine	1994
Wyeth (Wyeth Ayerst)	pneumococcal 7-valent conjugate vaccine	2000
Merck & Co. (Merck, Sharpe, and Dohme)	pneumococcal vaccine polyvalent	1977
Wyeth (Lederle Laboratories)	pneumococcal vaccine polyvalent	1979
Wyeth (Wyeth-Lederle)	poliovirus vaccine live oral trivalent	1963
Wyeth (Wyeth-Lederle)	poliovirus vaccine live oral type I	1962
Wyeth (Wyeth-Lederle)	poliovirus vaccine live oral type II	1962
Wyeth (Wyeth-Lederle)	poliovirus vaccine live oral type III	1962
Hollister-Stier Laboratories	polyvalent bacterial vaccines	1999
Wyeth (Wyeth-Ayerst)	rabies vaccine	1982
Chiron (Behringwerke)	rabies vaccine	1997
Bioport Corporation	rabies vaccine adsorbed	1998
Merck & Co.	rubella and mumps virus vaccine live	1970
Merck & Co.	rubella virus vaccine live	1969
Bioport Corporation	tetanus toxoid adsorbed	1998

TABLE 5-1 Continued

Company	Generic Name	U.S. Approval Date
Wyeth (Wyeth-Lederle)	typhoid vaccine	1952
Merck & Co.	varicella virus vaccine live	1995
Bioport Corporation (Michigan Department of Public Health)	anthrax vaccine adsorbed	1970
Wyeth (Wyeth Laboratories, Inc.)	cholera vaccine	1952

NOTE: Includes vaccines with active licenses that are not in production, e.g., cholera, plague, and oral polio vaccines.
SOURCE: Tufts Center for the Study of Drug Development, 2002.

COST STRUCTURE[1]

The costs of vaccine production include research and development (R&D) costs; costs related to the regulatory approval process; ongoing regulatory costs; plant costs, including depreciation; marketing costs; variable costs for labor, production, equipment, and supplies; and liability costs (Arnould and DeBrock, 2002).

Although there are substantial differences between development costs for vaccines and pharmaceuticals, the latter provide a useful benchmark. It has been estimated that, between 1980 and 1984, R&D and the regulatory approval process generated an average of 11 years of negative cash flow for NCEs introduced in the U.S. pharmaceutical industry (Grabowski and Vernon, 1997). DiMasi et al. (1991) estimate the mean out-of-pocket cost for a successful NCE at $32 million in 1987 dollars; when discovery, clinical testing, and failure costs are included, this figure rises to $115 million, while the inclusion of time and interest costs results in an estimate of $231 million (more than $300 million in 1997 dollars) (Grabowski

---

[1] Information on the costs and revenues associated with vaccine production is difficult to discern from the public record. The committee sought this information as part of its fact-finding effort by commissioning background papers on the vaccine industry (Arnould and DeBrock, 2002; Fine, 2003; Lichtenberg, 2002), corresponding with the five companies that produce recommended vaccines for the U.S. market (Aventis Pasteur, GlaxoSmithKline, Merck, Powderject, and Wyeth), inviting testimony in committee meetings from vaccine representatives, and condusting private interviews with company officials. This process yielded a substantial amount of qualitative information in support of the committee's analysis of the relationships among costs, revenues, returns, and investment in research and development (R&D). But verifiable, quantitative information on costs, revenues, and profits is lacking; and this lack of information represents an important limitation of this study.

TABLE 5-2 Foreign Producers of Vaccines for the U.S. Market

Company	Country	Generic Name	U.S. Approval Date
Statens Serum Institut	Denmark	diphtheria toxoid	1998
Statens Serum Institut	Denmark	tetanus and diphtheria toxoids	1998
Statens Serum Institut	Denmark	tetanus toxoid	1998
Aventis (Pasteur Merieux Connaught)	France	acellular pertussis DTP	1992
Aventis (Aventis Pasteur)	France	Bacillus Calmette-Guerin (BCG) live vaccine	1990
Aventis (Aventis Pasteur))	France	BCG vaccine	1998
Aventis (Aventis Pasteur)	France	conjugated haemophilus influenza b and diphtheria, tetanus, and acellular pertussis vaccine	1993
Aventis (Aventis Pasteur)	France	tetanus, diphtheria, polio and pertussis (cPDT) vaccine	2002
Aventis (Aventis Pasteur)	France	diphtheria and tetanus toxoids and pertussis vaccine adsorbed	1978
Aventis (Aventis Pasteur)	France	diphtheria and tetanus toxoids adsorbed	1984
Aventis (Aventis Pasteur)	France	diphtheria and tetanus toxoids adsorbed	1997
Aventis (Aventis Pasteur)	France	diphtheria and tetanus toxoids adsorbed, for adult use	1978
Aventis (Aventis Pasteur)	France	haemophilus B conjugate vaccine	1987
Aventis (Aventis Pasteur)	France	haemophilus b conjugate vaccine (tetanus toxoid conjugate)	1993
Aventis (Aventis Pasteur)	France	haemophilus b conjugate vaccine/diphtheria, tetanus toxoids, acellular pertussis vaccine in combination	1996
Aventis (Aventis Pasteur)	France	influenza virus vaccine	1978
Aventis (Aventis Pasteur)	France	meningococcal polysaccharide vaccine, group A	1978
Aventis (Aventis Pasteur)	France	meningococcal polysaccharide vaccine, group C	1978
Aventis (Aventis Pasteur)	France	meningococcal polysaccharide vaccine, groups A, C, Y and W-135 combined	1981
Aventis (Aventis Pasteur)	France	pertussis vaccine	1978
Aventis (Aventis Pasteur)	France	poliovirus vaccine inactivated	1987
Aventis (Aventis Pasteur)	France	poliovirus vaccine inactivated	1990
Aventis (Aventis Pasteur)	France	rabies vaccine	1980
Aventis (Aventis Pasteur)	France	rabies vaccine	1991
Aventis (Aventis Pasteur)	France	smallpox vaccine	1978
Aventis (Aventis Pasteur)	France	tetanus toxoid	1943

TABLE 5-2 Continued

Company	Country	Generic Name	U.S. Approval Date
Aventis (Aventis Pasteur)	France	tetanus toxoid	1978
Aventis (Aventis Pasteur)	France	tetanus toxoid adsorbed	1978
Aventis (Aventis Pasteur)	France	yellow fever vaccine	1978
Takeda Chemical Industries, Ltd.	Japan	acellular pertussis vaccine concentrate	1991
Research Foundation for Microbial Diseases	Japan	japanese encephalitis virus vacine inactivated	1992
Akzo Nobel (Organon Teknika Corp.)	Netherlands	BCG vaccine	1989
Cheil Jedang	South Korea	hepatitis-B vaccine	1988
Berna Sa (Swiss Serum and Vaccine Institute)	Switzerland	tetanus toxoid adsorbed	1970
Berna Sa (Swiss Serum and Vaccine Institute)	Switzerland	typhoid vaccine live oral	1989
GlaxoSmithKline (Smith Kline Beecham Biologicals)	UK	diphtheria and tetanus toxoids and acellular pertussis vaccine adsorbed	1997
GlaxoSmithKline (Smith Kline Beecham Biologicals)	UK	hepatitis A Inactivated and Hepatitis B (recombinant) vaccine	2001
GlaxoSmithKline (Smith Kline Beecham Biologicals)	UK	hepatitis B vaccine (recombinant)	1989
GlaxoSmithKline (Smith Kline Beecham Biologicals)	UK	hepatitis-A vaccine, inactivated	1995
Powderject Pharmaceuticals (Medva Pharma)	UK	influenza virus vaccine	1998
Statens Serum Institut	Denmark	diphtheria toxoid	1998
Statens Serum Institut	Denmark	tetanus and diphtheria toxoids	1998
Statens Serum Institut	Denmark	tetanus toxoid	1998
Aventis (Pasteur Merieux Connaught)	France	acellular pertussis DTP	1992

NOTE: Includes vaccines with active licenses that are not in production, e.g., pertussis monovalent and hepatitis B-Cheil Jedang vaccines.
SOURCE: Tufts Center for the Study of Drug Development, 2002.

and Vernon, 1997). A more recent study by DiMasi indicates that the out-of-pocket cost of an NCE has escalated to \$403–\$802 million (2000 dollars) when the time lag between investment and market release is capitalized (DiMasi et al., 2003).

Total development costs of bringing a vaccine to market are roughly similar to those for drugs and can be higher (Grabowski and Vernon, 1997). As part of the initial approval process, the FDA requires that the vaccines used in Phase III clinical trials be produced in a facility that will be used for commercial production if the vaccine is approved. As a result, manufacturers must frequently invest more than $30 million in the production facility prior to product approval (Grabowski and Vernon, 1997). Vaccine development costs have also risen as a result of the increased time it takes to achieve licensure, as well as larger FDA-required Phase III clinical trials for many recent vaccines (see Box 5-1). The size of clinical trials depends on a number of variables (Foulkes and Ellenberg, 2002), including the rates of disease and anticipated adverse events. The average size of clinical trials has increased over time (as has been the case for drugs) to provide an adequate base for identifying rare adverse effects during vaccine development. One industry expert estimates that a new vaccine costs $700 million from initial research to commercial production (Clarke, 2002). In addition to the requirement for early facility investments, production facilities for vaccines tend to be more capital-intensive than those for pharmaceuticals. On the other hand, vaccines tend to have higher success rates than pharmaceuticals and may be characterized by faster development times (Grabowski and Vernon, 1997).

Once a vaccine has been approved, the production process involves high fixed costs relative to variable costs. Fixed production costs, exclusive of up-front R&D and sales labor, represent 60 percent of total production costs for vaccines (Mercer Management Consulting, 2002). These fixed costs are not affected by changes in production volume. They are associated primarily with quality assurance activities, administrative labor, depreciation, and other manufacturing overhead. Industry representatives have indicated that increased regulatory requirements have resulted in increased costs for quality assurance employees relative to production employees. Semivariable costs make up 25 percent of total costs, excluding R&D and sales labor. Semivariable costs are batch costs that are constant per batch regardless of the number of batches (Mercer Management Consulting, 2002). Specific examples of batch costs are test animals and labor for production and testing. The remaining, variable, costs account for only 15 percent of total costs; examples of such costs are vials, stoppers, labels, packaging, and in-source components.

The costs of producing licensed vaccines have increased over the last decade as a result of several factors: mandatory removal of the mercury-containing preservative thimerosal, increased burdens associated with regulatory enforcement, a variety of improvements in vaccines that have been incorporated into existing products, both voluntary and mandated upgrading of production facilities, and increased direct provider shipment costs under new CDC contract arrangements (Hay and Zammit, 2002). Modern vaccines are also subject to constant updating and improvement, such as new stabilizers and new production technologies, as a result of

BOX 5-1
Vaccine Development and Approval

Vaccine development begins with basic research, which is usually conducted by universities, biotechnology firms, or pharmaceutical companies. Two government agencies—the National Institutes of Health (NIH) and the Food and Drug Administration (FDA)—also play particularly important roles, conducting or funding basic research that leads to or improves the development of vaccines, as well as providing advice to industry on the conduct and design of clinical trials. In addition, the FDA is responsible for vaccine licensure—the regulatory aspects of vaccine development and approval (Centers for Disease Control and Prevention [CDC], 2002j; CDC, 2002k).

To develop a vaccine for the U.S. market, the sponsor must first conduct preclinical trials, testing the proposed product in cell or tissue cultures and then in animals (CDC, 2002i). If preclinical studies indicate that the vaccine is potentially safe and effective, the sponsor files an independent new drug (IND) application with the FDA, requesting permission to test the vaccine in humans. The IND describes the vaccine, the manufacturing process, quality control testing, safety and immunogenicity data from animal trials, and the proposed protocol for clinical (human subject) trials (CDC, 2002i). A 30-day review period follows the filing of the IND. At the end of 30 days, unless otherwise notified by the FDA, the sponsor can begin the first of three sequential phases of clinical trials (Sing and Willian, 1996). The focus of each phase is as follows (CDC, 2002i; Sing and Willian, 1996):

• Phase I studies usually involve a small number of subjects (20–80) who are carefully monitored in tests of safety and immunogenicity.
• Phase II studies are generally conducted on several hundred subjects and are used to obtain additional data on immune response and adverse effects, including optimal dose ranges.
• Phase III studies typically involve several thousand subjects, providing more definitive data on the safety and efficacy of the vaccine.

Once Phase III clinical trials are at or near successful completion (i.e., the vaccine is deemed to be safe and efficacious), the sponsor submits two additional license applications seeking approval to manufacture and distribute the vaccine: a biologics license application (BLA), which licenses the vaccine; and an establishment license application (ELA), which licenses the facility where the vaccine is produced. During this phase of licensure, the sponsor provides a detailed accounting of the processes by which the vaccine is to be mass produced, as well as a description of how safety and efficacy will be documented on an ongoing basis. This phase also includes the FDA's detailed, on-site review of production facilities (CDC, 2002i; Sing and Willian, 1996).

Finally, some vaccines also undergo a postlicensure fourth phase of clinical trials to evaluate safety and effectiveness in the general population and to provide information on rare adverse events. Postlicensure trials generally include 100,000 or more subjects (Sing and Willian, 1996).

SOURCE: Adapted from Fine, 2003.

scientific advances. The MMR vaccine that is currently produced for the U.S. market is far different from the version produced in 1971, having been subject to an array of technical improvements (Arnould and DeBrock, 2002).

While the costs of producing vaccines have generally been increasing, the revenues from vaccine sales have remained relatively constant. The revenue potential of vaccines is limited by the small number of vaccinations usually required. Many prescription drugs are taken by patients for years; most vaccines are administered between one and four times over a lifetime. Furthermore, vaccine production costs do not necessarily decline over time. A key factor that contributes to higher production costs is the rigid batch inspection process, which makes it difficult for companies to achieve more efficiency through a learning curve and to enjoy cost reductions related to process improvements (Grabowski and Vernon, 1997). Pressures on revenues have resulted from CDC's ability to negotiate discounted federal contract prices, federal price caps on certain vaccines since 1993, the gradually increasing public share of vaccine purchases (at discounted prices), and the addition of price competition to the government contracting process. The principal exceptions to this revenue picture relate to two fairly new vaccines—varicella and pneumococcal conjugate—which are priced higher than earlier vaccines.

RESEARCH AND DEVELOPMENT

In 2000, the leading global vaccine companies spent about $750 million on R&D (Mercer Management Consulting, 2002). This figure is significantly smaller than the $26.4 billion allocated to pharmaceutical R&D worldwide (Arnould and DeBrock, 2002). The United States has been responsible for the discovery and development of two-thirds of the world's new vaccines in the last 20 years. The major contributors to vaccine research in the United States are companies conducting industrial research, government agencies (the National Institutes of Health [NIH] and the Department of Defense [DoD]), and the academic institutions they fund.

There were 285 vaccine R&D projects ongoing in 1996 (not including HIV vaccine efforts), of which 133 were in the clinical trials phase (Grabowski and Vernon, 1997). Mercer Management Consulting (2002) reports that this activity had increased by 2000 to nearly 350 R&D projects—188 in the pre–clinical trial phase and 158 in clinical trials. The rate of U.S. approval of vaccine licenses has also been increasing. Between 1997 and 1999, 17 new licenses were approved, compared with 8 licenses between 1990 and 1992 (Mercer Management Consulting, 2002). A recent IOM study identifies additional vaccines that are expected to be developed by 2010 (IOM, 2000b) (see Box 5-3).

Industrial Research

The National Vaccine Advisory Committee (NVAC) estimates that vaccine sales financed 46 percent of the $1.4 billion spent on vaccine R&D in 1995 (CDC, 1997). Vaccine R&D is conducted by both large and small companies. Large companies spent an estimated 15 to 20 percent of their product sales—about $650 million—on R&D in 1995. Many small biotechnology firms, ranging in size from 36 employees (Antex Biologics, Inc.) to over 1,600 employees (Immunex Corporation), are also involved in vaccine research. Their total sales range as well, from $500,000 (AVAX Technologies, Inc.) to almost $1 billion (Immunex Corporation). In 1995, small companies invested $250 million in vaccine R&D (CDC, 1997).

Some biotechnology firms receive funding directly from the government to develop vaccines for the military, such as vaccines against diarrhea and gastroenteritis. Other firms are subsidiaries of larger pharmaceutical companies or may be partially owned by another firm. Many small vaccine start-up companies receive a significant portion of their funding through venture capital (Arnould and DeBrock, 2002).

Some firms focus solely on vaccine research, while others emphasize multiple approaches to a single type of disease. Major targets of current research include respiratory diseases, viral hepatitis, sexually transmitted diseases (STDs), herpes virus diseases, parasitic diseases, fungal infections, and cancer vaccines. A recent breakthrough in research on the human papilloma virus (HPV) holds the promise of eliminating cervical cancer (Schultz, 2003). Vaccines in the pipeline, including recombinant vaccines for HIV, herpes simplex, diabetes, and infertility (see Box 5-2), are increasingly complex (Mercer Management Consulting, 2002).

One of the major areas of recent research is vaccines for STDs and vaccines that can be effective in children. Extensive effort has been focused on finding a vaccine for HIV to stop the worldwide spread of the virus. Scientists have learned a great deal about how the immune system works through this research. This knowledge has spurred research on cancer vaccines, and the market for such vaccines is projected to grow significantly through 2007.

R&D projects are frequently aimed at diseases for which vaccines are not yet available (see Table 5-3). But a substantial amount of research is also directed toward vaccines that would be improvements upon or combinations of existing licensed vaccines, as well as directly competing vaccines. Considerable research is also directed toward new methods for administering vaccines, such as the recently FDA–approved nasal spray form of influenza vaccine (FDA, 2003).

Despite these signs of commercial interest, product development is increasingly costly relative to the market potential of vaccines. The ab-

BOX 5-2
Vaccines Expected to Be Developed by 2010

Borrelia burgdorferi
Chlamydia
Coccidioites immites
Cytomegalovirus
Enterotoxigenic *E. coli*
Epstein Barr
Human papilloma virus
Helicobacter pylori
Herpes simplex
Histoplasma capsulatum
HIV
Hepatitis C
Influenza
Insulin-dependent diabetes mellitus (therapeutic)
Melanoma (therapeutic)
Multiple sclerosis
Mycobacterium tuberculosis
Neisseria gonorrhea
Neisseria meningitidis B
Para influenza
Respiratory syncytial virus
Meningococcus
Rheumatoid arthritis (therapeutic)
Rotavirus
Shigella
Streptococcus group A
Streptococcus group B

SOURCE: IOM (2000b) (HIV added).

sence of a market capable of supporting production costs and providing an adequate return on investment, for example, has hampered the development of vaccines for malaria and other diseases that affect primarily the developing world (Kremer, 2000b). In 2000, the Global Alliance for Vaccines and Immunization (GAVI) was founded in part to respond to the need for vaccines in developing countries. GAVI is also interested in improving technologies for administering vaccines in the difficult environments commonly found within developing countries.

TABLE 5-3 Deaths from Selected Diseases Not Yet Preventable by Immunization

Disease	Deaths (000)	%
AIDS	2,285	27.5
Tuberculosis	1,498	18.
Malaria	1,110	13.
Rotavirus	800	9.6
Shigella	600	7.2
Enterotoxic E. coli	500	6.0
Respiratory syncytial virus	160	1.9
Schistosomiasis	150	1.8
Leishmaniasis	42	0.5
Trympanosomiasis	40	0.5
Chagas disease	17	0.2
Dengue	15	0.2
Leprosy	2	0.0
Total deaths	8,319	100.0

SOURCE: Arnould and DeBrock, 2002, adapted from Kremer, 2000a.

Government Support

The government is involved in vaccine R&D in numerous ways. Among the federal entities supporting R&D, the most important is NIH, which is responsible for identifying and supporting the development of potential vaccines. The FDA oversees the regulatory process for bringing a new vaccine to market. The CDC is the largest single buyer and distributor of vaccines in the United States. DoD conducts its own research on vaccines and supports research at academic institutions, focusing primarily on vaccines for military and bioterrorism applications. The U.S. Agency for International Development (USAID) has a limited role in supplying vaccines to other countries, largely by providing grants to institutions in the developing world.

The government encourages investment in R&D through a combination of push and pull strategies. Push programs involve the use of public resources to support research, whereas pull programs reward the developer after a project has been successfully completed.

The most important push strategy is funding of vaccine research by NIH, which is responsible for approximately one-third of all vaccine research funding (Arnould and DeBrock, 2002). Although some NIH research is conducted internally, most of the work on vaccines is supported through grants to academic institutions and health-related agencies. The

National Institute of Allergy and Infectious Diseases (NIAID) is the primary vaccine research entity within NIH. NIAID funding for basic vaccine and bioterrorism research in 2002 was $2.4 billion. NIH allocates about 60 percent of its funds to basic research, with the remainder supporting clinical trials. In 1988, NIH provided an estimated 14 percent of all funding for preclinical pharmaceutical R&D and 11 percent of funding for clinical trials (Arnould and DeBrock, 2002).

The most salient pull strategy employed by the government is the use of patents to protect property rights, which encourages R&D in many areas, including vaccines (Kremer, 1998). Patents are awarded to an individual or firm that establishes legal proof of original discovery and generally prohibit anyone but the patent holder from marketing the product for a period of 17 years from the patent award date. With a guaranteed period of market exclusivity, the patent holder can capture monopoly profits that subsidize the R&D costs involved in obtaining the patent and compensate for the expensive regulatory hurdles related to safety and efficacy.[2] Absent patent protection, competitors would simply imitate or reverse-engineer the product without paying for the original R&D costs and charge a marginal-cost price shortly after marketing approval, eroding the originator's profits and substantially diminishing the incentives for innovation. Moreover, under the patent system, the monopolist is rewarded with profits in the market that are roughly proportional to market demand and societal willingness to pay. This solves the other problem involved in rewarding innovation: how the government or the public can determine or monitor what a patent is actually worth.

While patent protection treats vaccines and drugs in a similar fashion, some have argued that patents are not as relevant in vaccine development (Arnould and DeBrock, 2002). The reasoning is that other barriers to competitive entry—such as the long production start-up cycle, the level of business risk, the monetary investment required to achieve product and plant licensure, and the steep learning curve with respect to regulatory oversight—are of greater importance than patents in sustaining the production of vaccines.

Further, as with pharmaceuticals, an increasingly stringent process for clinical trials and FDA approval can reduce the effective patent life of a vaccine product.[3] The patent system also has economic limitations.

---

[2]Patents may sometimes be awarded for different vaccine products that are close substitutes, as is sometimes the case with pharmaceutical products. In these cases, monopoly profits may not be obtained.

[3]To encourage the marketing of drugs that may have been patented long before potential FDA approval, the Waxman Hatch Act guarantees a minimum of 5 years of exclusive marketing to the patent holder for any FDA-approved pharmaceutical.

Patents restrict output and raise prices, which means that some consumers will not benefit from vaccines that are under patent. Many patients who would be willing to pay the competitive price of vaccines, and more, will forego monopoly-priced vaccines.

Another pull strategy is to subsidize or otherwise increase prices (Kremer, 2000a). The margin by which prices exceed costs—including investment in R&D and production costs—determines profitability, and also finances new R&D and sends a signal to the industry about future returns that can be expected from current investments (Grabowski and Vernon, 1997).

To a certain extent, the government's strategies for stimulating R&D are blunted by the length and cost of the FDA regulatory process that is designed to foster safe and effective products. Furthermore, the extent of government purchasing power in the marketplace has held prices down, reducing incentives for R&D. As noted by Kremer (2000a), even if vaccine manufacturers received full market price on every dose sold, vaccines would still remain socially undervalued; that is, the price that individual buyers in a competitive market would be willing to pay would be less than the price society would be willing to pay for the benefit derived from vaccines.

INDUSTRY CONCENTRATION

The rate of concentration in the vaccine industry has increased over the last four decades. Between 1966 and 1977, half of all commercial vaccine manufacturers stopped producing vaccines; and the exodus continued into the 1980s and 1990s. Between 1967 and 1980, the number of manufacturers licensed to produce vaccines for the U.S. market dropped from 26 to 17 (Cohen, 2002). Of the nine producers leaving the U.S. market during this period, eight were domestic firms (Sing and Willian, 1996).

These declines have continued in recent years. By 1996, a total of eight firms and laboratories were producing recommended childhood vaccines for the U.S. market (Sing and Willian, 1996). In 2002, only four firms remained (GAO, 2002). Similar exits have occurred among manufacturers of adult vaccines. The most recent of these was Wyeth's discontinuation of its influenza and pneumococcal polysaccharide vaccines (Wyeth Pharmaceuticals, 2002).

Three major factors influenced structural changes in the U.S. vaccine market from the mid-1960s through the early 1980s: (1) new FDA regulations, starting in 1972, that required evaluation of all previously licensed biological products (rather than submit data for evaluation, many firms simply withdrew from the market and requested that FDA revoke their licenses "without prejudice"); (2) growing concerns about liability; and

(3) poor returns on investments relative to pharmaceutical and other products in the corporate portfolio (IOM, 1993). More recent observers have cited underlying economic reasons—particularly selected aspects of the cost structure of vaccine production relative to the size of the U.S. market—for the small number of suppliers in the U.S. childhood vaccine market. An analysis by Grabowski and Vernon (1997) focuses on four such factors: regulatory costs, liability costs, R&D costs, and low risk-adjusted returns relative to pharmaceutical products. Other observers of the recent decline in the number of producers of U.S. childhood vaccines have cited similar factors in market departures, including new safety-related requirements (removal of the mercury-containing preservative thimerosal), regulatory compliance issues, and investment decisions based on the larger portfolio of parent companies (GAO, 2002; Orenstein, 2002a).

The diminishing number of vaccine manufacturers has reduced the number of vaccine products within the U.S. market. Of the 146 vaccines approved since 1933, 62 were subsequently withdrawn from the market (see Table 5-4). Some withdrawals represent replacement decisions, whereby an approved vaccine was replaced by a more effective or safer product. The diphtheria–tetanus–whole-cell pertussis (DTP) vaccine, for example, was replaced by the safer acellular pertussis version, DTaP. (Box 5-3 illustrates trends in the supply of DTaP.) Combination vaccines have also been introduced, replacing "single-indication" vaccines in vaccination schedules. Much current R&D and product testing is directed toward expansion of combination vaccines because they generally reduce the number of doses and the administration costs of vaccination, even though they may be more expensive (Ellis and Douglas, 1994; see also Chapter 3).

What is more troubling is the effect of economic factors on the withdrawal of vaccine products that are viewed as unprofitable or yield low returns relative to the production of pharmaceutical products. In some cases, demand for older vaccines is not strong enough to warrant continued production.[4] Another reason for exit arises when the costs of vaccine operation and regulatory compliance are too great to support more than one producer. Often the result can be one or two suppliers, or no supplier, of the entire specific vaccine segment, as is the case with the vaccine for indicators of Lyme disease.

The changing structure of the U.S. vaccine industry reflects an international trend. As noted earlier, five multinational producers dominate global vaccine sales, although many small foreign producers exist as well.

---

[4]The producer of a vaccine for Lyme disease, for example, pulled out of the market because of inadequate product demand.

TABLE 5-4 Approved Vaccines Withdrawn from the U.S. Market

Company	Country Name	Generic Name
Merck & Co. (Merck, Sharpe, and Dohme)	United States	tetanus toxoid
Wyeth (Lederle)	United States	staphylococcus toxoid
Eli Lilly	United States	tetanus toxoids
Bayer Corp. (Cutter)	Germany	tetanus toxoid
Pfizer (Parke, Davis and Co.)	United States	tetanus toxoid
Merck & Co. (Merck, Sharpe, and Dohme)	United States	typhus vaccine
Wyeth (Lederle)	United States	cholera vaccine
Bayer Corp. (Cutter)	Germany	plague vaccine
Wyeth (Lederle)	United States	Rocky Mountain spotted fever vaccine
Wyeth (Wyeth Laboratories)	United States	smallpox vaccine (vaccinia)
Wyeth (Wyeth-Lederle)	United States	tetanus toxoid
Merck & Co. (Merck, Sharpe, and Dohme)	United States	influenza virus vaccine
Pfizer (Parke, Davis and Co.)	United States	influeza virus vaccine
Pfizer (Parke, Davis and Co.)	United States	diphtheria and tetanus toxoiuds and pertussis vaccine adsorbed
Bristol-Myers Squibb (E.R. Squibb)	United States	6-valent pneumococcal vaccine
Eli Lilly	United States	diphtheria and tetanus toxoids
Merck & Co.	United States	diphtheria and tetanus toxoids and pertussis vaccine adsorbed
Pfizer (Parke, Davis and Co.)	United States	diphtheria and tetanus toxoids
Wyeth (Lederle) antitoxin	United States	gas gangrene polyvalent
Merck & Co. (Merck, Sharpe, and Dohme)	United States	cholera vaccine
Pfizer (Parke, Davis and Co.)	United States	diphtheria and tetanus toxoids and pertussis vaccine
Wyeth	United States	diphtheria toxoid adsorbed
Pfizer (Parke, Davis and Co.)	United States	poliomyelitis vaccine
Pfizer (Parke, Davis and Co.)	United States	adenovirus vaccine
Delmont Laboratories	United States	polyvalent bacterial antigens
Pfizer (Parke, Davis and Co.)	United States	adenovirus and influenza vaccines combined aluminum phosphate adsorbed
Pfizer	United States	Polio vaccine, live, oral Type 1
Pfizer	United States	Polio vaccine, live, oral Type 2
Pfizer	United States	Polio vaccine, live, oral Type 3
GlaxoSmithKline (Glaxo Wellcome)	United Kingdom	BCG vaccine

continued

TABLE 5-4 Continued

Company	Country Name	Generic Name
Merck & Co. (Merck, Sharpe, and Dohme)	United States	typhoid vaccine
Pfizer (Parke, Davis and Co.)	United States	diphtheria, tetanus toxoids, pertussis vaccine absorbed, poliomyelitis vaccine
Merck & Co. (Merck, Sharpe, and Dohme)	United States	smallpox vaccine
Wyeth (Lederle)	United States	measles vaccine
Aventis (Aventis Pasteur)	France	smallpox vaccine
Merck & Co. (Merck, Sharpe, and Dohme)	United States	measles-smallpox vaccine, live
Wyeth (Lederle)	United States	typhus vaccine
Wyeth (Lederle Laboratories)	United States	diphtheria and tetanus toxoids and pertussis vaccine adsorbed
Wyeth (Wyeth Laboratories)	United States	diphtheria and tetanus toxoids adsorbed
Wyeth (Wyeth Laboratories)	United States	diphtheria and tetanus toxoids adsorbed for adult use
Wyeth (Wyeth Laboratories)	United States	diphtheria and tetanus toxoids adsorbed
Wyeth (Wyeth Laboratories)	United States	diphtheria and tetanus toxoids adsorbed for adult use
Wyeth (Wyeth Laboratories, Inc.)	United States	diphtheria and tetanus toxoids and pertussis vaccine adsorbed
Wyeth (Lederle)	United States	tetanus toxoid adsorbed

SOURCE: Tufts Center for the Study of Drug Development, 2002.

As a result, five of the current recommended vaccines in the United States have only one producer, and the others have either two or three. Prior to the 1980s, vaccine markets had regional, not global, leaders. Pasteur-Merieux and SmithKline led the European market, Merck and Lederle-Praxis were major suppliers for the U.S. market, and three Japanese firms (Takeda, Eisai, and the Research Foundation of Osaka University) were the major suppliers for the Japanese market. By the early- to mid-1990s, global acquisitions, mergers, and joint ventures had reshaped the industry as a whole (Mowery and Mitchell, 1995).

The decline in the number of vaccine producers reflects the consolidation that is occurring within the pharmaceutical industry as a whole. But it is also driven by the decisions of pharmaceutical companies to drop vaccines from their product portfolios. A rash of such exits occurred in

---

BOX 5-3
Vaccine Supply: The Case of DTaP

The supply of the diphtheria-tetanus-acellular pertussis (DTaP) vaccine provides a good example of trends for the industry as a whole. Key trends include the following.

The total number of firms producing DTaP for the U.S. market has declined. While five DTaP vaccines have been licensed in the United States since 1991, only three are currently being produced; and of these, two are produced by subsidiaries of the same multinational corporation, Aventis Pasteur. Companies have left the market for many reasons, including concerns about product liability lawsuits, investments required to enhance production quality, and the anticipated costs of removal of the mercury-based preservative thimerosal.

The portion of the market represented by U.S.-based firms has not just diminished but been reduced to zero. Of the five firms originally licensed by the Food and Drug Administration (FDA) to produce DTaP, two (Lederle and North American Vaccine) had corporate headquarters in the United States. Today, all three DTaP vaccines currently on the U.S. market are produced by two European-based corporations: GlaxoSmithKline and Aventis-Pasteur (which produces both Tripedia and Daptacel).

Finally, the corporate history of the five DTaP vaccines licensed in the United States reflects both the astounding number of acquisitions and mergers that have taken place within the industry and the extent to which these activities have concentrated the production of relatively expensive vaccines in the hands of very large American or European multinational corporations. Of the five vaccines licensed in the United States to date, only one, approved in May 2002, is still produced by the same company—Aventis Pasteur, Ltd., a Canadian subsidiary of French-based Aventis Pasteur. Of the remaining companies originally licensed to produce DTaP in the United States, all have undergone one or more mergers or acquisitions since licensure; and all have become part of major multinational corporations.

SOURCE: Adapted from Fine, 2003.

---

the 1980s as a result of growing concern about liability exposure. In response, Congress passed the National Childhood Vaccine Injury Act in 1986, a no-fault damage award system designed to compensate victims who experienced adverse consequences from vaccine products, as well as to protect companies from litigation that might disrupt the production of vaccines with social benefits. Recently, litigation over thimerosal, an ethyl mercury-containing vaccine preservative, has raised questions about the effectiveness of the vaccine injury award system. The use of novel legal theories designed to circumvent the National Childhood Vaccine Injury Act is a source of deep concern to the industry (GlaxoSmithKline, 2002; Merck, 2002; Pisano, 2002).

The rate of exit from the vaccine industry raises two chief concerns. The most immediate of these is the lack of backup capacity should a manufacturer experience production problems or other disruptions. When Wyeth opted out of the production of DTaP in 2000, for example, the suddenness of the firm's withdrawal left competing firms unable to fill the gap, resulting in a 2-year shortage of the vaccine. Production efforts by other companies to compensate for such a supply disruption can take well over a year (Pisano, 2002). Longer-term concerns include the potential for the exercise of market power by the remaining firms and the potential for the total loss of supply of a vaccine product.

Industry observers have consistently issued warnings about the threats posed by the sole-supplier situation and the potential for supply interruptions given the existence of single producers of many vaccines, including 10 of the 15 recommended childhood vaccines (DeBrock and Grabowski, 1985; Arnould and DeBrock, 1993). The number of producers continues to decline as the number of vaccines provided by a single supplier increases (see Table 5-5) (CDC, 2003g).

REGULATION

Safety review is the responsibility of the FDA's Center for Biologics Evaluation and Review (CBER). Careful monitoring for purity and quality is required for vaccines, which are produced from or use living cells and organisms, as well as complex growth materials taken from living sources. Subtle changes in materials, process, or environment alter the final vaccine product and can affect its safety or effectiveness. Each batch must be carefully tested for composition and potency through a batch release process. Unlike other drugs, vaccines are used on healthy people to prevent disease; and as a result, vaccine production is subject to higher standards of safety than is the case for pharmaceuticals (Crawford, 2002).

Vaccine manufacturers have stated that while the regulatory guidelines (Current Good Manufacturing Practices) governing the production of vaccines have not changed substantially over the last decade, significant shifts have occurred in the interpretation and intensity of enforcement of those guidelines by CBER (Merck, 2002; Pisano, 2002). In a presentation to the committee, one industry representative illustrated this situation using a metaphor from baseball: "It's not that the strike zone has

TABLE 5-5 Number of Producers of Selected
Vaccines for the U.S. Market, 2003

Vaccine	Number of Producers
Haemophilus influenzae type b	3
Influenza	2
Hepatitis A	2
Hepatitis B	2
Diphtheria and tetanus toxoids and acellular pertussis (DTaP)	2
Measles–mumps–rubella (MMR)	1
Tetanus toxoid	1
Tetanus–diphtheria[a]	1
Inactivated poliovirus	1
Varicella (chickenpox)	1
Pneumococcal conjugate (PCV-7)	1
Meningococcal	1
Pneumococcal polysaccharide (adult)	1

[a]A small amount of Td is produced by the Massachusetts Public Health Biological Laboratories.
SOURCE: CDC, 2003g.

changed; it's the way it's called." According to the vaccine producers, the
new approach to enforcement reflects limited knowledge of vaccine
manufacturing processes and important differences between pharmaceutical and vaccine facilities. Even minor changes in packaging may require
a complete product review and relicensing of a vaccine production facility.

The FDA can also change requirements suddenly. Thimerosal is a
good example (Freed et al., 2002b). Although levels of ethyl mercury did
not exceed accepted guidelines, the FDA in 1999 required the removal or
reduction of thimerosal in all pediatric vaccines. This decision necessitated major changes in production and bottling processes, including the
replacement of multidose vials with single-dose vials that have different
fill-volume requirements. Estimates of the impact of this change on product losses range from 20 to 30 percent for certain vaccines (Aventis Pasteur, 2002).

PRICING

Substantial variations occur in vaccine pricing that reflect the volume
of sales and the market power of the buyer. As a general rule, most individual clinicians, clinics, and hospitals pay list price or near list price to

purchase vaccines. Large group purchasing organizations, state consortia, and health plans can negotiate discounts of up to 15 percent (Mercer Management Consulting, 2000).

The federal government has historically negotiated discounts of 40–50 percent below list price, although the discounts have been lower for the most recent vaccines. Federal contract prices averaged 75 percent less than catalog prices in 1987 and 50 percent lower in 1997 (IOM, 2000a). In contrast, discounts for varicella and pneumococcal conjugate vaccines were 9 and 22 percent, respectively, in 2002 (Orenstein, 2002b). Box 5-4 presents details on the vaccine purchasing practices of the Veterans Administration and DoD.

The committee identified two significant concerns with regard to vaccine prices. First, as noted earlier, the prices of new vaccines are very high relative to those of older vaccines, and these higher prices present significant problems for federal and state health budgets, clinicians, and consumers. Immunization rates may decrease when costs become too burdensome to the payor. The second concern is that some vaccine prices are too low and do not encourage desirable levels of investment in R&D and production capacity. Federal contracts for several vaccines are subject to price caps that have held price increases to no more than the rate of inflation since 1994. The price cap has been cited in particular as the major obstacle to the negotiation of a government contract for the tetanus toxoid vaccine. Detailed historical prices are shown in Table 5-6; trends in vaccine prices in current (2002) dollars are illustrated in Figure 5-1.

Vaccine price trends fall into four distinct periods.[5] Up to and during most of the 1970s, vaccine prices were comparatively low and stable. Prices even decreased slightly for many vaccines during the 1970s.

The second period began in 1982, when prices increased sharply and continued to rise until the early 1990s. For example, an increase of 2,847 percent in the price of DTP occurred during the 15-year period 1977–1991 (IOM, 1993).

The third period occurred during the 1990s, when prices tended to be stable and in some cases declined. However, new vaccines appeared on the market, in some cases (e.g., inactivated poliovirus [IPV] and DTaP) replacing older vaccines at higher prices. For example, the DTaP contract price of $11.01 in 1992 was almost double the DTP price of $5.99.

The fourth period, characterized by the introduction of new vaccines at dramatically higher prices, began in the mid-1990s with the release of the varicella vaccine at a federal contract price of $32.70 per dose. This new pricing model continued with the introduction in 2000 of the new

---

[5]This discussion is based on price data supplied by CDC (2002l; 2003d).

BOX 5-4
Vaccine Purchasing by the Veterans Administration and the
Department of Defense

Veterans Administration

The VA purchases vaccines using the federal supply schedule (FSS) for pharmaceutical and biological products. The FSS was established as part of the VA Health Care Act. Its purpose is to limit the prices paid for drugs and vaccines by placing a cap on prices that can be paid by the federal government. The FSS price cap is established each January and is based on 73 percent of the average nonfederal price. Companies may then set an FSS price at or below the price cap. They can also change their price at different times throughout the year, as long as they remain under the cap. Some FSS prices—e.g., for hepatitis A and B vaccines—are typically set below the price cap; others are set at the cap. There has been no CDC contract for adult pneumoccocal vaccine for the last several years because no company will sell below the FSS cap.

CDC does use the FSS in establishing maximum prices for adult vaccines: hepatitis A and B, pneumoccocal polysaccharide, and tetanus-diphtheria. One company challenged CDC's use of the FSS for varicella in nonfederal facilities, and the Department of Health and Human Services supported CDC. The matter is still a point of contention. The FSS is not used for childhood vaccines because the Vaccines for Children (VFC) legislation superceded the VA Health Care Act's authority for these vaccines. There is no relationship between CDC contract prices and FSS prices, and CDC contract prices are often higher (e.g., varicella).

FSS prices therefore apply to only a small fraction of vaccines purchased—those purchased for use by the Department of Defense (DoD) and the VA and state purchases of adult vaccines. But a general relationship exists between the FSS and private-sector vaccine prices, because the FFS cap is a fixed percentage of private-sector prices.

Department of Defense (DOD)

DoD purchases vaccines for military use by troops, but also for routine care for service personnel and their dependents. Vaccines are purchased by the Pharmaceuticals group of the Defense Supply Center in Philadelphia, using competitive contracts common in military procurements.

SOURCE: IOM, 2002g.

TABLE 5-6 Federal and Private Prices of Vaccines Per Dose, 1983–2002 (nominal prices, excise taxes excluded)

Year	Td		Hib		Hepatitis B	
	Federal	Private	Federal	Private	Federal	Private
1983						
1984	0.08					
1985	0.08					
1986	0.08					
1987	0.08					
1988	0.15		11.00	13.75		
1989	0.09		6.00	13.75		
1990	0.81		4.80	14.55	7.66	
1991	0.09		5.16	14.55	7.43	
1992	0.12		5.34	15.28	7.13	
1993	0.11	0.83	5.32	14.82	7.11	
1994	0.13	1.00	4.20	15.25	7.34	16.17
1995	0.13	1.00	4.76	15.13	7.68	17.09
1996	0.13	1.00	4.98	15.13	7.91	17.59
1997	0.13	NA	4.55	14.07	8.06	16.84
1998	0.14	1.00	4.73	15.40	8.36	20.09
1999	No contract	2.50	4.36	15.67	8.25	23.74
2000	No contract	NA	4.45	15.67	8.27	24.42
2001	No contract	NA	5.19	15.67	8.25	21.54
2002	No contract	NA	6.70	15.67	8.55	21.54
2003	No contract	NA	7.76	18.98	8.5	22.95

pediatric pneumococcal vaccine at $43.50 per dose (the list price was $58.00). Prices of older vaccines, on the other hand, have remained stable, despite considerable new investment in upgrading of facilities and the removal of thimerosal. However, the recent stability of pricing for older vaccines may be disrupted by the development of new combinations of individual vaccines and of existing vaccine combinations. For example, GlaxoSmithKline recently received approval for its DTaP–IPV–Hepatitis B combination. The initial list price of this new vaccine is only a few dollars higher than the sum of the prices of the separate vaccines, but the long-term pricing strategy for such new combinations is not yet clear.

The increase in the public share of vaccine purchases also affects prices. Because of deep government discounts, the expanding public market for vaccines results in lower average prices for their manufacturers. In addition, when contracting for the purchase of vaccines, the Veterans Administration (VA) penalizes firms for increasing prices charged to its nongovernment customers. For any increase in price higher than the con-

Hepatitis A		Varicella		PCV-7		Pneumococcal Conjugate	
Federal	Private	Federal	Private	Federal	Private	Federal	Private
						3.24	NA
						2.94	NA
						2.94	NA
						2.94	NA
						2.92	NA
						3.21	NA
						3.37	10.03
						3.35	7.66
						3.24	8.17
11.17	11.17					No contract	8.17
11.15	28.45	32.70	41.41			No contract	8.17
11.08	28.45	33.65	40.66			3.72	9.12
11.75	24.49	33.65	40.98			3.80	9.57
11.18	25.17	34.66	43.51			5.46[a]	NA
11.15	27.45	36.39	44.81	44.02	58.00	5.61[a]	NA
11.15	27.45	38.39	44.81	45.24	58.00	No contract	NA
11.15	NA	40.69	44.81	45.24	58.00	No contract	NA
11.28	29.68	43.33	57.36	47.5	58.75	No contract	NA

continued

sumer price index, the VA reduces the allowable Federal Supply Schedule (FSS) price that can be paid under federal contract. This practice has resulted in FFS vaccine prices as low as $0.01 per dose.

SHORTAGES

Over the past 20 years, the nation has experienced two major periods of vaccine supply shortages. The first was related to the product liability crisis of the mid-1980s, when production of DTP vaccine was curtailed as a result of manufacturers leaving the U.S. market. The second period of supply shortages lasted from fall 2000 to summer 2002. During this period, the United States experienced nationwide shortages of five childhood vaccines that protect against eight of the eleven childhood diseases prevented through routine immunization (GAO, 2002) (see Table 5-7). The recent shortages affected most of the manufacturers of childhood vaccines,

TABLE 5-6 Continued

Year	MMR Federal	Private	OPV Federal	Private	IPV Federal	Private
1983	4.70	11.30	0.58	3.56		
1984	5.40	12.08	0.73	4.60		
1985	6.85	13.53	0.86	6.15		
1986	8.47	15.15	1.68	8.67		
1987	6.32	17.88	1.14	8.07		
1988	12.23	19.67	1.07	7.78		
1989	12.23	19.67	1.63	9.11		
1990	10.27	19.63	1.63	9.45		
1991	10.89	20.85	1.71	9.11		
1992	10.89	20.85	1.80	9.62	7.30	NA
1993	10.89	16.41	1.87	9.85	7.52	14.38
1994	11.25	20.85	1.92	10.18	7.48	14.67
1995	11.56	21.43	1.98	10.18	4.99	14.67
1996	11.87	25.56	2.03	10.18	5.20	14.67
1997	12.12	27.75	2.08	10.18	5.46	14.67
1998	12.33	23.33	2.11	10.18	5.79	14.67
1999	12.44	25.21	2.15	10.18	6.04	14.67
2000	12.83	25.94	Replaced by IPV		7.00	14.67
2001	13.28	25.94			7.50	14.67
2002	13.39	25.94			8.05	14.67
2003	13.74	32.48			9.21	21.78

NA = Not Available

[a]Adult vaccine only, since there was no contract for the childhood vaccine because of the price cap.
NOTE: All prices represent the lowest-price packaging option for each supplier. For 1992

with three of the four experiencing supply problems during the period (Orenstein, 2002b).

Supply problems were especially severe for vaccines that are in continuous demand, such as those for tetanus and influenza. In March 2000, there were two major producers of tetanus vaccine in the United States—Aventis Pasteur and Wyeth-Ayerst—and no shortages. By early January 2001, Wyeth had ceased production of the vaccine, leaving Aventis as the only supplier.[6] Aventis could not scale production up rapidly enough to

---

[6]Brichacek (2001) indicates that the Wyeth pullout from manufacturing the tetanus vaccine may have been related to a June 2000 issue with the FDA concerning acellular pertussis vaccine.

DTP		DTaP		Influenza	
Federal	Private	Federal	Private	Federal	Private
0.42	0.45				
0.65	0.99				
2.21	2.80				
3.01	11.40				
3.13	8.92				
3.90	6.47				
3.40	6.09				
2.35	6.09				
1.69	5.41			1.03	NA
1.43	5.41	6.45		No contract	1.82
1.33	5.48	5.37	6.97	No contract	1.82
1.41	NA	5.42	11.53	No contract	NA
Replaced by DTaP		5.71	11.27	1.72	NA
		9.50	11.27	1.53	NA
		8.28	14.63	1.61	NA
		7.05	14.69	1.54	2.15
		7.00	14.69	2.14	2.15
		7.00	14.72	2.37	NA
		8.34	15.33	4.41	NA
		9.87	15.56	5.53	5.00
		10.31	17.40	5.53	6.50

and later, prices indicated are weighted averages based on the number of doses ordered at each price (calculations by the IOM committee). Previous years' averages supplied by CDC. SOURCE: CDC, 2002l, 2003d.

meet demand and was forced to ration supply (Arnould and DeBrock, 2002).

Several of these shortages were severe enough that the Advisory Committee on Immunization Practices (ACIP) recommended suspension of booster doses for tetanus–diphtheria (Td), DTaP, and pneumococcal conjugate. Shortages were most severe for Td and pneumococcal conjugate, for which there was a 40 percent shortfall in doses shipped. Shipments of varicella decreased by 26 to 29 percent. The stockpile of MMR was drawn down by 700,000 doses, but shipments were still off by 15 percent (Orenstein, 2002a). There were delays in adult influenza vaccine in the two previous seasons, and severe shortages of tetanus toxoid affected the availability of doses for adult boosters and emergency use. By July 2002, these shortages, with the exception of pneumococcal conjugate, had

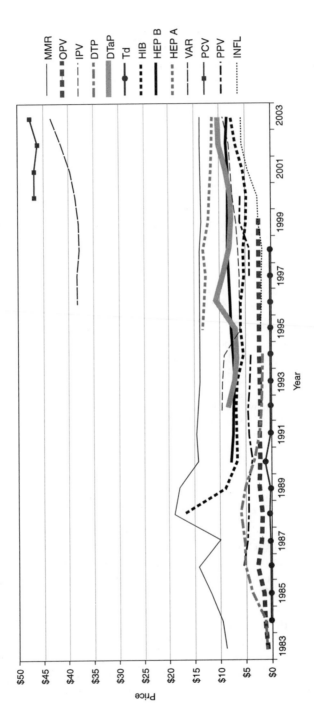

FIGURE 5-1 Federal contract vaccine prices in current dollars.
NOTE: PPV = pneumococcal polysaccharide vaccine.
SOURCES: CDC, 2002l, 2003d.

TABLE 5-7 Vaccine Supply Status in 2001–2002

Supply Problems	No Supply Problems
• Tetanus–diphtheria • DTaP • MMR • Varicella (chickenpox) • Pneumococcal 7 valent (PCV- 7)	• *Haemophilus influenzae* type b (Hib) • Hepatitis B • IPV • Hepatitis A • Meningococcal polysaccharide • Influenza • Adult pneumococcal

SOURCE: Orenstein, 2002c.

ended; supplies of pneumococcal conjugate vaccine are expected to return to normal in 2003 (CDC, 2003h).

No reports of regional outbreaks of preventable infectious diseases occurred during this period of vaccine shortages. However, shortages place stress on the fragile public–private partnership that delivers vaccines to the public. Public compliance with the recommended schedule can be threatened by the lack of vaccines and sudden changes in the schedule resulting from shortages. CDC reports that, as a result of the tetanus vaccine shortage, 52 percent of states suspended school immunization laws (Orenstein, 2002a). Given the recent intensity of antivaccine rhetoric, school administrators find themselves in an uncomfortable role as enforcers of laws that they themselves may not adequately understand. In a recent poll of school nurses, the majority of respondents indicated their belief that children may be receiving too many vaccines (Lett, 2002). These trends may make it difficult to reinstate school laws that are suspended as a result of shortages.

It is too soon to determine whether the recent shortages were a one-time event or an early sign of a recurring pattern. An important structural risk factor in supply disruption—the limited number of suppliers—has not changed. With only four suppliers for all universal childhood vaccines and monopoly suppliers of four of those vaccines, the United States remains highly vulnerable to disruptions in manufacturer production.

Vaccine shortages appear to result from specific and apparently unrelated causes rather than a single overriding factor (GAO, 2002; NVAC, 2003) (see Table 5-8). Vaccines affected by the shortages are both new, such as pneumococcal conjugate, and long-standing, such as MMR; and shortages have affected both sole-supplier and multiple-supplier vaccines. Some explanations for the shortages that have been advanced by the industry include problems associated with removing thimerosal from the production process, compliance with increasingly stringent Current Good

TABLE 5-8 Vaccine Shortages and Their Causes

Vaccine	Immediate Cause of Shortage	Shortage Period
DTaP	Two producers withdrew in 2000: Baxter acquired North American Vaccine and withdrew its DTaP product. Wyeth withdrew as of January 2001. The two remaining suppliers, GSK and AvP, had insufficient capacity to supply full demand. AvP experienced production slowdowns due to the removal of thimerosal.	4th quarter 2000 to 3rd quarter 2002
Td	In January 2000, Wyeth withdrew from production of tetanus vaccine.	4th quarter 2000 to 3rd quarter 2002
MMR	Merck, the sole producer, interrupted production to address issues related to Current Good Manufacturing Practices. 700,000 doses were borrowed from the stockpile.	January 2001 to July 2002
Varicella	Production ceased from September 2001 to November 2001 because of scheduled modifications to production facilities, which took longer than expected.	4th quarter 2001 to 2nd quarter 2002
Pneumococcal conjugate	Unexpectedly strong demand overwhelmed supply, combined with a January 2002 production bottleneck.	October 2001 to present
Influenza	Multiple manufacturers had difficulty growing one of the flu strains, combined with increased demand due to a recommendation change (reduction in the age of the primary target group from 65 to 50) and quality control issues at Parkdale and Wyeth.	2000–2001 flu season
	Vaccine production was delayed; only two-thirds of the supply was available by October.	2001–2002 flu season

SOURCES: DTaP and Td: Fine, 2003; other: Mason, 2002.

Manufacturing Practices, disruptions due to plant renovations, unanticipated high demand for new vaccines, and sudden withdrawals from the market by producers. The FDA licensure process may create a structural barrier to rapid adjustment of output to address sudden shortfalls in supplies. The agency's requirement for full-scale production capacity before licensure is granted may tend to fix minimal excess capacity at start-up. Combined with the stringent entry requirements and lead times for licensure, little flexibility to adjust production remains (Arnould and DeBrock, 2002). There is also evidence that other developed countries, while not experiencing the critical shortages of the United States, are characterized by capacity constraints that could lead to shortages (Mercer Management Consulting, 2002).

Some have sought a relationship between vaccine pricing and shortages (Orenstein, 2002c). As shown in Table 5-9, however, short-run correlations between vaccine prices and shortages are not apparent. Prices for vaccines with supply problems are generally higher than those for vaccines without such problems. A more meaningful relationship would involve profit margins, yet even this relationship may be confounded by other variables.

STOCKPILES

The vaccine stockpile program consists of an inventory system of storage and rotation contracts negotiated with manufacturers. Initiated in 1983 to establish a 6-month strategic reserve of each universally recommended vaccine, the program was initially funded with Section 317 funds. By 1988, stockpiles had been developed for six important vaccines and combinations (DTP, tetanus toxoid [TT], Td, oral poliovirus [OPV], IPV, and MMR). The Omnibus Budget Reconciliation Act (OBRA) of 1993 allowed VFC federal entitlement funds to be used for stockpile purchases, but approval from the Office of Management and Budget (OMB) is required for this purpose. CDC began to target purchases toward vaccines with sole suppliers to minimize financial risk. Multiple withdrawals from the stockpiles occurred between 1984 and 2002, mainly as a result of temporary

TABLE 5-9 Vaccines With and Without Supply Problems (2002)

With Supply Problems			Without Supply Problems		
Vaccine	Contract Price	Catalog Price	Vaccine	Contract Price	Catalog Price
Td	[a]	$7.50 avg. state	IPV	$8.25	$15.42
DTaP	$10.58–$10.65	$17.12	Hib	$5.75–$8.00	$15.25–$18.95
MMR	$15.53	$28.35	Hep. B	$9.00	$21.40–$24.20
Varicella	$39.14	$49.13			
PCV-7	$45.99	$58.75			

[a]Price capped at $0.144; no contract could be negotiated.
SOURCE: Orenstein, 2002c.

manufacturing problems. The most recent drawdown was 700,000 units of MMR in 2001 (see the discussion of shortages, above). Of ten vaccines that CDC has targeted for stockpiling, only three were stockpiled in 2002 (Lane, 2002).

Building up the stockpiles to full strength and possibly increasing their capacity could help alleviate the shortages discussed earlier (GAO, 2002). Rebuilding the stockpiles would require substantial investment and OMB clearance. GAO has also recommended legislation that could authorize the use of VFC stockpiles for non–VFC-eligible recipients in cases of national shortage. But even at full strength, the stockpile program provides only a temporary buffer in cases of serious supply disruption. Given the time required for licensing a new facility and ramping up production, the stockpiles would be inadequate in the face of a total manufacturer withdrawal. No government contingency plan exists for this prospect.

Stockpiles are also costly. Moreover CDC has been conservative about developing stockpiles to minimize financial risk from, for example, a change in vaccine recommendations that could render a stockpile useless. Examples of such changes include the switch from OPV to IPV, the elimination of thimerosal from certain vaccines, and the future replacement of individual and exisiting combination vaccines with new combinations.

CDC CONTRACTING

Each year, CDC negotiates a federal contract for the purchase of ACIP-recommended childhood vaccines. CDC does not directly purchase vaccines; state and local grantees are each given a vaccine budget for the purchase of vaccines at the negotiated contract prices. With that budget, states can purchase, store, and redistribute these vaccines from their own depots or through contracts with pharmaceutical distribution companies. Some states allow clinicians to choose among competing vaccine products. States can also purchase vaccines under the CDC contract for non-VFC vaccines for other federally authorized state programs. Of the 52 percent of vaccines purchased under the federal contact, 35 percent are for the VFC program, while the remaining 17 percent are purchased by states using both Section 317 funding (10 percent) and state funds (7 percent) (Orenstein, 2002b).

Several factors in addition to negotiating leverage determine the contract prices. For some vaccines (OPV, IPV, *Haemophilus influenza* type b, Hib, MMR, DTP, DTaP, Td, adult pneumococcal, and hepatitis B), there are statutory price caps that were imposed at the time VFC was enacted to prevent rapid escalation of prices. The price caps hold vaccines to their price on May 1, 1993, plus an annual inflation adjustment. DTaP and hepatitis B are no longer subject to the cap. Vaccines that were approved after the enactment of the VFC program have never been subject to a cap. These include hepatitis A, influenza, varicella, and pneumococcal conjugate (CDC, 2002m).

Vaccine companies do not always bid the maximum price of the cap. For example, Merck has always bid the maximum for MMR, while Aventis Pasteur has consistently bid below the cap for IPV, despite its monopoly on that product (CDC, 2002m).

CDC has also introduced competition into the contract design. The original "winner take all" contracts were initially replaced with a multiple-supplier contract that guaranteed the largest market share to the lowest bidder (all Section 317 and half of VFC purchases). In 1998, CDC introduced the current competitive approach, under which states can purchase from the supplier of their choice at the federal contract price. Manufacturers can attempt to increase their market share by lowering their price several times during the contract period.

Private-sector buyers purchase vaccines through both wholesale distributors and direct customer sales. Clinicians typically pay high prices to distributors, but they are able to make small purchases when needed and benefit from business relationships with local distributors (Mercer Management Consulting, 1995).

In contrast with childhood vaccines, the public sector purchases a very limited share of adult vaccines. For example, only about 2 percent of the 90 million doses of trivalent influenza vaccine sold in the United States in a single year is purchased through federal contracts (Johnson, 2002). The two U.S.-based manufacturers of influenza vaccine emphasize direct sales to end users instead of to distributors.[7] The third manufacturer is based in the United Kingdom and relies on U.S. distributors. Also, bulk-purchase arrangements are common with adult vaccines. Many employers offer mass vaccination services in the workplace. One large mass vaccinator recently reported administering over 1 million doses during the 2001–2002 influenza season. Premier, a group purchasing association representing about one-third of the hospital beds in the United States, contracts for several million doses of influenza vaccine for its members each year (CDC, 2002n).

BARRIERS TO A WELL-FUNCTIONING
VACCINE SUPPLY SYSTEM

This chapter has identified a number of barriers to a well-functioning vaccine supply system. These barriers are reviewed in turn below.

---

[7]One of the two domestic producers recently dropped out of the influenza vaccine market.

Exit and Concentration

Concerns about the possibility of a total loss of supply of a critical vaccine are widespread. These concerns have spawned national debate and research on the reasons for the apparent fragility of vaccine supplies. For example, NVAC has held numerous discussions of and recently released a report on vaccine supply (NVAC, 2003). The Council of the IOM also issued a statement in 2001 calling for the creation of a national vaccine authority to address this problem (IOM, 2001).

However, exit of manufacturers from vaccine production and the resultant concentration of supply cannot, by themselves, be considered a system failure. For example, substantial economies of scale combined with a limited U.S. market may mean that only one efficient producer can survive for each vaccine. But recent vaccine shortages suggest that the industry may not be able to produce a stable supply under current conditions.

Research and Development

Maintaining a vital R&D enterprise has been a cornerstone of U.S. vaccine policy and the basis for patent regulations and NIH research funding. Yet research has suggested that significant disparities exist between private incentives to invest in R&D and the social benefits of vaccines (Kremer, 2000a,b). Additional public support may be necessary to address these disparities if the full potential of vaccines as valuable tools of disease prevention is to be achieved. As Kremer further points out, however, R&D depends on the expectation of firms that they will be adequately rewarded for their investment. Too many aspects of vaccine policy in the United States—including government pricing polices, licensure requirements, and regulation—send negative signals to companies. While regulation and reasonable pricing are each important, achieving national policy goals requires that they be balanced and coordinated. There are many indications that the opposite is in fact the case.

Barriers to Entry

Perhaps the most important long-run solution to the fragility of vaccine supplies is to ensure that multiple companies have access to the U.S. market. Although a large number of small domestic R&D firms and foreign companies have applications pending for vaccine licenses in the United States, regulatory and cost barriers may inhibit the entry of many of these producers. For example, a company that has had a successful vaccine product in use for many years in Europe and Canada must conduct full clinical trials as part of its U.S. license application rather than drawing on efficacy and safety data from its current product experience. GAO (2002) has recommended expedited FDA review procedures. Implementing this recommendation would accelerate approval of new and competitive vaccines in the case of shortages and also reduce the total cost of bringing a vaccine to market.

Regulation

FDA product and facility regulations are important to the safety of the vaccine supply and the viability of the industry. According to industry experts, however, the impact of regulation has been costly, without clear evidence of corresponding improvements in quality (GlaxoSmithKline, 2002; Merck, 2002). A government planning authority does not exist at a high enough level that can balance national objectives of safety, as embodied in the FDA's regulation of production, and availability, which depends in part on the regulatory burden faced by vaccine producers.

Undervaluation of Vaccines

Industry representatives frequently allude to the role of federal pricing policies as evidence of the undervaluation of vaccines. They suggest that the elimination of vaccine-preventable diseases has reduced the perceived threat of those illnesses and also decreased the perceived value of vaccines. Although substantial research has demonstrated the social benefits of vaccines, economic analysis suggests that vaccines are persistently undervalued (IOM, 2000b; Kremer, 2000a). The increased costs of newer vaccines—such as pneumococcal conjugate at $176,000 per quality-adjusted life-year saved—has changed the picture dramatically. As a result, it is no longer possible to generalize across all vaccines in discussing social valuation.

Several proposals have been offered to reduce the gap between the social value and price of vaccines. McGuire (2003) proposes a method for setting an administered price of a vaccine according to its social benefit (see Box 6-2 in Chapter 6). In McGuire's formulation, a preset price is determined that maximizes consumer surplus subject to profit maximization of the producing firm, based on an estimate of the social benefit of the vaccine. Putting this approach into practice would depend on the existence of estimates of the average benefit of a vaccine. A recent IOM report (IOM, 2000b) presents a cost-effectiveness analysis of 26 candidate vaccines, applying a common analytical framework for measuring the costs and effects of vaccine development and administration. Other authors have used a similar framework. Kremer (2000a) estimates that in the developing world, a vaccine against malaria would be cost-effective at

$41 per dose; but that under the current purchasing system for developing countries, producers would probably receive only around $2 per dose, which is too low to stimulate appropriate investment.

On the other hand, it is clear that the prices of newer vaccines, such as pneumococcal conjugate and varicella, are considerably higher than those of their predecessors. This situation may reflect higher costs, higher profits, or both. Given the vaccine industry's recent pricing trends, undervaluation is a phenomenon that applies principally to older, routine vaccines.

FINDINGS

The amount that the nation spends on vaccines appears to be insignificant compared with that spent on other medical and social interventions that may have lesser social benefits. While federal and state governments must address the vaccine line item as an expense to be managed, a commitment of resources substantially higher than current levels may be justified to address persistent breakdowns in the vaccine system.

The relationship between financial returns to the vaccine industry and future investment in production capacity and R&D is a fundamental concern addressed by this study. While proprietary industry information was not available to the committee, a large body of indirect and secondary evidence suggests that high development and production costs and stable revenues have constrained investments in new products within the vaccine industry as a whole. While many new candidate vaccines are in early stages of development, the overall level of investment in vaccine products is too low to support the level of R&D that is desirable in light of the social benefits of immunization. The committee finds that

- The U.S. vaccine market is small relative to total expenditures on personal health services and pharmaceuticals. The entire global market for vaccines is roughly equivalent to the sales of certain individual blockbuster drugs.
- The supply of U.S. vaccines is becoming highly concentrated, resulting in limited backup capacity in the event of supply disruptions.
- Inadequate build-up of vaccine stockpiles has limited their remedial effect on recent shortages. The development of 6-month stockpiles would help avert short-term disruptions in supply but would not address more fundamental concerns, such as the continuing loss of suppliers from the industry.
- The risks and costs to manufacturers associated with vaccine production have increased. Key factors include regulation, removal of the preservative thimerosal, and an increase in vaccine injury lawsuits.

- FDA resources for vaccine regulation have not kept pace with the growth and complexity of vaccine products. FDA regulation has shifted from a focus on science to a focus on enforcement. This shift may increase the risks and costs associated with vaccine production without increasing safety.

- The pace of vaccine R&D, particularly in the discovery stage, is currently high, but commercial development is impeded by pricing and industry returns. Investment in production capacity for existing vaccines is especially problematic.

- FDA licensure requirements—including the increasing size of clinical trials, the requirement that companies build full production capacity before licensure, and the inadmissibility of clinical data from outside the United States for U.S. licensure—create substantial barriers to entry.

- The requirement for building full plant capacity in advance of approval may limit fixed capacity and increase the chances of shortages.

- Vaccine company investments in R&D on new vaccines are sensitive to prices and expected returns on investment. Ensuring socially desirable levels of R&D may necessitate prices that are substantially higher than current prices for most routine childhood vaccines.

- By using its bargaining power to achieve substantial discounts in federal contracts, CDC may substantially undervalue vaccines and reduce industry incentives for investment in both R&D and short-run production capacity.

Summary of Conclusions

Conclusion 1: Current public and private financing strategies for immunization have had substantial success, especially in improving immunization rates for young children. However, significant disparities remain in assuring access to recommended vaccines across geographic and demographic populations.

Conclusion 2: Substantial increases can be expected to occur in public and private health expenditures as new vaccine products become available. While these cost increases will be offset by the health and other social benefits associated with these advances in vaccine development, the growing costs of vaccines will be increasingly burdensome to all health sectors. Alternatives to current vaccine pricing and purchasing programs are required to sustain stable investment in the development of new vaccine products and attain their social benefits for all.

Conclusion 3: Many young children, adolescents, and high-risk adults have no or limited insurance for recommended vaccines. Gaps and fragmentation in insurance benefits create barriers for both vulnerable populations and clinicians that can contribute to lower immunization rates.

Conclusion 4: Current government strategies for purchasing and assuring access to recommended vaccines have not addressed the relationships between the financing of vaccine purchases and the stability of the U.S. vaccine supply. Financial incentives are necessary to protect the existing supply of vaccine products, as well as to encourage the development of new vaccine products.

Conclusion 5: The vaccine recommendation process does not adequately incorporate consideration of a vaccine's price and societal benefits.

6

Conclusions and
Alternative Strategies

The preceding chapters of this report have highlighted key issues related to the history and organization of vaccine finance in the United States, as well as the many factors that influence vaccine access and availability. This chapter reviews those prior discussions and summarizes the committee's conclusions. It also describes the alternative strategies the committee considered in formulating the recommendations presented in Chapter 7.

In developing its conclusions and recommendations, the committee sought to devise a set of financing strategies that could achieve the twin goals of (1) assuring access to recommended vaccines and (2) sustaining the availability of vaccines in the future. At present, these two goals are addressed through a fragmented system of separate programs: payments by some private health care insurance plans (which distribute the costs to consumers and employers through premiums), personal out-of-pocket payments, public vaccine purchase programs (such as Vaccines for Children [VFC] and state universal purchase programs), and public health care finance arrangements (such as Medicare). Government efforts to assure access to recommended vaccines have evolved incrementally and in separate policy arenas. The cumulative impact of these efforts is that federal purchases now exceed 50 percent of the childhood vaccine market through the VFC and Section 317 programs. The government pricing strategy has focused on obtaining deeply discounted vaccine prices.

These strategies have worked reasonably well in assuring access for children. Yet these same strategies have been blamed, in part, for reducing the financial incentives for private investment in the production and licensing of vaccines.[1] Firms have abandoned vaccine products or left the vaccine business completely, and unprecedented vaccine shortages occurred in 2001 and 2002. In addition, health care providers are increasingly concerned about the inability to recover payment for their costs of purchasing and administering vaccines to children and adults. Private-sector providers, who currently administer over 80 percent of childhood vaccines, continue to refer patients to public health clinics for vaccinations, creating missed opportunities that can delay or prevent immunization and reduce overall immunization rates for vulnerable populations. It is in this context that the committee presents the following conclusions, which in turn form the basis for the recommendations in Chapter 7.

CONCLUSIONS

The introduction of new vaccines in the coming decades will impose additional and sometimes unexpected financial burdens on public and private health care plans, providers, and consumers. These burdens are offset by the value of these new vaccines, including financial savings that result from decreased medical expenditures, enhanced quality of life, reduced care-giving burdens, and gains in productivity associated with the prevention of infectious disease.

Vaccines for contagious diseases have strong spillover effects, given that immunization interrupts the disease transmission process and reduces the likelihood that an infection will harm others. Current and potential new vaccines that protect against contagious diseases are the strongest candidates for public investments in vaccine assurance efforts, since the spillover effects of these vaccines are substantial (Pauly and Cleff, 1995). But not all future vaccines will have the same level of spillover effects. Some future vaccines will prevent specific noncontagious diseases, such as certain forms of cancer and immune system disorders, rather than inhibiting the spread of contagious disease (see Box 2-1 in Chapter 2). The committee views vaccines that do and do not have these spillover effects quite differently. There is a more compelling rationale for strong federal intervention in the case of vaccines with spillover effects, since they are the ones most likely to be undervalued in the market and therefore to require subsidization.

---

[1]The manufacturer removed the tetanus vaccine from the federal contract, claiming that the government price cap was too low to sustain its production. In presenting the fiscal year 2004 federal budget, President Bush proposed amendments to the VFC legislation to remove price caps; this action would allow the tetanus and diphtheria vaccine to be restored to the VFC program.

This distinction is viewed as increasingly important since the proportion of vaccines in the pipeline that do not address highly contagious diseases is growing. Although all vaccines share certain public-good properties in terms of basic research and development, the spillover effects in consumption of vaccines provides the key rationale for broad public support of vaccine financing. The rationale is less compelling in the case of vaccines without these spillover effects, except in certain cases where the public benefits of the vaccine are exceptionally high. Burdening the national immunization system with the financing of a new generation of expensive vaccines without substantial spillover effects would divert resources away from vaccines that benefit the public more broadly.

The committee sought to design financing strategies that could resolve the tensions among growing public-sector demand for vaccines; higher vaccine expenditures; and the economic incentives that influence the development, production, and administration of vaccines.

Conclusion 1: Current public and private financing strategies for immunization have had substantial success, especially in improving immunization rates for young children. However, significant disparities remain in assuring access to recommended vaccines across geographic and demographic populations.

Current efforts have not achieved the *Healthy People 2010* goal of immunizing 80 percent of all 2-year-old children. One in four young children is not up to date in receiving recommended immunizations. Sustaining current levels of immunization (about 74 percent) and achieving future immunization goals are threatened by predictable financial pressures in the coming decade as new and more expensive vaccines are added to the recommended schedule for children and adults.

Immunization rates for adults aged 65 and older have improved (66 percent for annual influenza and 50 percent for pneumococcal vaccine in 1999) since the inclusion of influenza and pneumococcal vaccines in Medicare benefits, and more than doubled in the period 1988–1995 (GAO, 1995). However, morbidity and morality rates for both diseases remain significant in this population. Immunization rates for high-risk adults aged 18–64 are especially poor. Most working-age adults with chronic illness (including such disorders as heart and lung disease and diabetes), who are at particular risk for vaccine-preventable disease, have not received the recommended immunizations. In 1999, only 31.9 percent received an annual influenza vaccination, while only 17.1 percent had ever received a pneumococcal vaccination (NCHS, 2000). The difficulties associated with risk-based strategies (i.e., based on health conditions) for adults have caused many providers within the health profession to shift to an age-based strategy. One example is the recent Advisory Committee on Immunization Practices (ACIP) guideline for influenza vaccine, which recommends immunization of all adults over age 50 (replacing the earlier guideline of 65 and older).

The relationships among cost barriers, access to recommended vaccines, and immunization status are uncertain. Immunization rates are highest among young children (aged 5 and under) and adults (aged 65 and older), who have the broadest access to vaccines through government-supported vaccine purchase programs. Immunization rates remain low among the high-risk adults aged 18–64 years, for whom no dedicated vaccine finance programs exist apart from those who are enrolled in Medicaid.

In addition to uneven immunization rates at the national level, substantial variation (almost 20 percent) in immunization rates currently exists within and across states. Some large urban centers, in particular, have difficulty achieving high immunization rates for children aged 19–36 months. The causes of these disparities are not well understood, but low levels of immunization are commonly associated with areas characterized by a concentration of poverty and groups that frequently move in and out of safety net programs. The disparities in vaccine-preventable disease burden between children and adults are especially troubling.

> **Conclusion 2: Substantial increases can be expected to occur in public and private health expenditures as new vaccine products become available. While these cost increases will be offset by the health and other social benefits associated with these advances in vaccine development, the growing costs of vaccines will be increasingly burdensome to all health sectors. Alternatives to current vaccine pricing and purchasing programs are required to sustain stable investment in the development of new vaccine products and attain their social benefits for all.**

Although the costs associated with purchasing and delivering vaccines have historically been small, new vaccines will be priced at higher levels reflecting the scale of investment necessary to bring new products through the licensing and production processes. The addition of new vaccines to the recommended schedule and the higher costs associated with newer vaccine products have placed tremendous stress on safety net programs that are already straining to achieve public health goals. Higher vaccine prices can be expected to exacerbate such problems as uneven distribution patterns, delays in the vaccine price negotiation processes for federal and state contracts, and continued fragmentation in the scope of vaccine benefits included in public and private health plans. An increased burden on public health clinics also occurs when private health plans reduce reimbursements for recommended vaccines in the face of higher costs. This burden places substantial stress on public health budgets and interferes with the ability to provide vaccines to traditional safety net populations, as well as those who lack vaccine benefits within their health plans.

It should be noted that vaccines provide a net long-term savings in health care costs. Over time, vaccines should lead to a diminution in what would otherwise be spent on health care. But certain sectors (such as state and federal health agencies) will bear substantial short-term costs of acquiring and delivering vaccines.

Increases in the budgets of government vaccine programs should be seen as acceptable, indeed desirable, insofar as new vaccines can offer substantial public health benefits. What is missing in the array of current vaccine purchasing programs is a clear and deliberate strategy that the government can use to stabilize and assure adequate rates of return on future private investments in vaccine development. While the true costs of innovation remain unknown, government pricing systems and bulk purchases alone appear to provide insufficient incentives, according to industry sources, given the higher production costs and uncertainties associated with vaccine development and the tendency to push down prices in the public sector.

Conclusion 3: Many young children, adolescents, and high-risk adults have no or limited insurance for recommended vaccines. Gaps and fragmentation in insurance benefits create barriers for both vulnerable populations and clinicians that can contribute to lower immunization rates.

Many individuals (referred to as "underinsured") have private health insurance that does not include coverage for vaccines. Estimates of underinsured children vary from 5 to 14 percent of all children. Others have insurance policies that require individuals to cover vaccine costs in the form of high deductibles and copayments. Still others, such as Medicare beneficiaries, are covered for certain vaccines but not others. Persons who face such financial barriers are less likely to receive routine immunizations in their medical homes and may fail to receive certain immunizations at all.

Although most large public and private health plans include vaccine benefits, signs of slippage are occurring within the scope of vaccine benefits offered by small businesses and other large subscribers, such as public employee health plans. The omission of or limitations on vaccine benefits in health plans, coupled with increasing deductibles and copayments, create gaps that existing safety net programs cannot easily fill. The result is increasing fragmentation and administrative barriers that interfere with the timely delivery of vaccines within routine health care services.

The multifaceted eligibility determinations associated with the current fragmented system of public and private vaccine benefits represent a serious barrier to immunization by imposing substantial burdens on physicians and other health care providers. Clinicians must determine whether the costs of purchasing and administering recommended vaccines are reimbursable under the terms of a wide variety of insurance plans and entitlements, including VFC, the State Children's Health Insurance Program (SCHIP), Section 317, Medicare, and multiple private health insurance plans. These administrative barriers can result in missed opportunities for immunization and frequent referrals of underinsured patients to public health clinics for routine vaccines, which in turn ultimately contribute to shortfalls in immunization rates.

Conclusion 4: Current government strategies for purchasing and assuring access to recommended vaccines have not addressed the relationships between the financing of vaccine purchases and the stability of the U.S. vaccine supply. Financial incentives are necessary to protect the existing supply of vaccine products, as well as to encourage the development of new vaccine products.

Tensions exist in the vaccine supply system between the need to control the current costs of vaccine purchases and the need to spend more money for innovation and the production of present and future vaccines. The desire to maximize short-term savings in purchasing current vaccine products and to maintain price caps is directly opposed to the goal of creating financial incentives for commercial firms to develop new vaccine products. Policy efforts to resolve recurring tensions among escalating vaccine costs, tighter health budgets, and the desire for sustainable and competitive markets in the vaccine industry have been limited to a series of stopgap measures and policy proposals in recent years (Fairbrother and Haidery, 2002). Thus, federal and state governments currently lack a coherent policy that can assure an appropriate balance among these objectives. The result is uncertainty among both producers and purchasers, which in turn reduces incentives for future vaccine development and threatens to exacerbate current disparities in immunization rates among insured, underinsured, and uninsured populations.

Conclusion 5: The vaccine recommendation process does not adequately incorporate consideration of a vaccine's price and societal benefits.

The recommendations of ACIP and its counterpart groups within the American Academy of Pediatrics and the American Academy of Family Physicians have significant implications for public and private expenditures. For example, ACIP recommendations directly affect vaccine prices and supply, such as the addition of vaccine products to the recommended vaccine schedule, the inclusion of vaccines in the VFC entitlement program, the standard of care for the Medicaid vaccine schedule, and the universal purchase guidelines for many states. Yet the ACIP decision-making process requires the formulation of recommendations before the government purchase price of a vaccine product is known. In addition, ACIP has no mechanism for distinguishing vaccines with strong spillover effects, such as those that prevent highly contagious diseases, from vaccines that do not, such as tetanus and therapeutic vaccines (such as cancer vaccines) that are in development. The lack of a capacity to address these variables is a serious impediment to a coherent finance strategy for vaccine purchases in the national immunization system.

ALTERNATIVE STRATEGIES

In framing its recommendations, the committee focused its analysis on seven alternative approaches, which included market-oriented, government intervention, and incremental strategies. Each approach was considered in terms of its impact on both access to vaccines and incentives for the production and development of vaccines in the private sector. In addition, the committee sought to design a strategy that would maintain a reasonable budget for vaccine purchases for children and adults in the public and private health sectors. The committee evaluated dozens of proposals for changes to the immunization system that had been developed by congressional committees, professional and industry associations, government agencies, advocacy groups, and experts before focusing its efforts on seven alternative strategies (including the current system).[2] Each proposal was considered in light of the following goals:

- Eliminate individual financial barriers to immunization.
- Increase incentives to the industry to invest in R&D and production capacity.
- Reduce provider burden and improve provider compensation.

---

[2]Some of these approaches were summarized in background papers prepared for the committee, including Fairbrother and Haidery (2002), Hay and Zammit (2002), and McGuire (2003). Others were included in recent reports on vaccine supply by GAO (2002) and NVAC (2003).

- Minimize fragmentation of financing and delivery.
- Maintain existing community and provider relationships.
- Control escalation of costs and increasing fiscal burden on state budgets.

There are several tensions among these objectives. For example, increasing incentives to industry, if achieved through higher prices, could conflict with controlling costs. Higher vaccine prices would also increase costs to providers, further fragmenting delivery, and to state budgets, thereby increasing fragmentation of financing. In addressing these conflicts, the question of increasing or decreasing government involvement emerges as a key factor. A universal government purchase program would address most of the above objectives. However, the committee views the growing share of government in vaccine purchasing as a discouragement to vaccine investment. Indeed, the committee determined that no single alternative can satisfy every objective; each involves trade-offs, assumptions, and perhaps ideological orientations. The following analysis of alternatives is meant to illuminate these trade-offs so they can be clearly understood. The final recommendation formulated by the committee combines elements of several different approaches to balance competing objectives.

The committee considered the following seven alternative approaches:

1. Maintain the current system.
2. Expand the VFC program to include additional eligibility categories.
3. Provide universal coverage through federal purchase and supply of all recommended vaccines.
4. Provide a federal block grant to the states for vaccine purchase.
5. Use public vouchers to purchase recommended vaccines for disadvantaged populations.
6. Create an insurance mandate that would require public and private health plans to cover all recommended vaccines.
7. Combine features of the insurance mandate and voucher alternatives into a new funded mandate system.

These approaches are described below, along with the merits and deficiencies of each. They are further summarized in Table 6-1.

Alternative 1: The Current System

Description/Design Options

The current system is based primarily on the VFC entitlement, which provides free vaccines to approximately 10 million safety net children through private office-based practices and community health centers. The program is supplemented by Section 317 grants to states and state-funded programs. Through VFC, the federal government assures access to the vaccines that prevent 11 diseases[3] for certain categories of children (aged 0–18): all uninsured and Medicaid-eligible children, Native Americans and Alaska Natives; and children who receive recommended vaccines in federally qualified health centers (FQHCs).[4] The federal government also assures access to vaccines against influenza and pneumonia for all adults over age 65 through the Medicare program. In addition, younger adults (aged 18–64) who receive Medicaid benefits have access to certain vaccines if recommended by their physician as part of a treatment plan.

Vaccines are purchased under a federal contact negotiated by CDC for the states on behalf of the eligible populations of children and adults. VFC does not include provider fees, which are typically paid with Section 317 or state funds. Program growth will result from the increasing numbers of the eligible population (mainly uninsured and Medicaid children), the addition of new vaccines that are likely to be recommended for children in the next two decades, and higher prices of new vaccines.

Advantages

There are some advantages to maintaining the current system. In nearly a decade of experience, VFC has been successful in enhancing public insurance coverage among children and improving their immunization rates. Public health advocates have indicated that the presence of a federal entitlement has provided stable and certain funding not subject to the fiscal budgetary pressures faced by discretionary programs.

---

[3]Diphtheria, tetanus, pertussis, measles, mumps, rubella, polio, *haemophilus influenzae* type b, hepatitis B, varicella (chickenpox), and invasive pneumococcal disease.

[4]The VFC entitlement was initially restricted to FQHCs. In January 2003, President Bush announced his intention to seek legislation that would amend the VFC legislation to include all state and local health clinics as access sites (U.S. Department of Health and Human Services, 2003).

TABLE 6-1 Summary of Alternative Strategies for Vaccine Purchases

Features	1. VFC (Current System)	2. Expanded VFC	3. Universal Federal Purchase
Description	Federal entitlement that provides free vaccines to participating public and private providers. CDC purchases vaccines for distribution to the states.	Continuation of central features of VFC entitlement. Expands VFC to include immunization of underinsured children in other health care settings (not just FQHCs).	Federal government purchases all recommended vaccines and gives vaccines to states for distribution to providers. Replaces VFC and state purchases. Providers/insurers may not charge patients for the free vaccines. Requires that all insurers cover administration fees for recommended vaccines, with some level of discretion.
Eligibility	Children (aged 0–18) who are • Medicaid-eligible • Uninsured • American Indian or Alaska Native • Receive vaccines in FQHCs.	All children eligible for VFC; *plus* all underinsured children, regardless of health care setting; *plus* all uninsured and underinsured adults with high-risk health conditions, regardless of health care setting.	All children and adults.

4. Federal Block Grant	5. Public Vouchers	6. Insurance Mandate	7. Funded Mandate
In lieu of vaccine, states receive federal funds for immunizations (amounts based on amount of current VFC purchases).	Health care providers purchase vaccines for uninsured persons and receive reimbursement from the federal government.	All public and private health plans are required to reimburse health care providers for costs of all recommended vaccines.	All public and private health plans are required to reimburse health care providers for replacement costs of all recommended vaccines.
States allocate federal funds to support immunization efforts (e.g., vaccine purchase, infrastructure investment, and special programs).	Voucher pays providers a fixed amount for immunization (payment to cover purchase cost and administration fee for each vaccine).	Insurers must report levels of vaccine coverage and cost-sharing fees to the federal government.	Health plans receive payment from the federal government to cover vaccine costs and provider fees on a periodic basis.
States must meet federally determined immunization goals (state-specific) or face penalties or loss of the grant.	Federal government sets amount of voucher for each vaccine based on a calculation of social benefit.	Applies only to vaccines that have low coverage rates 5 years or more after being introduced (e.g., more than 5% of target population remains uninsured for the vaccine).	Voucher subsidy is used for uninsured patients.
			Health plans and providers can keep the difference between the subsidy and the actual vaccine purchase price.
Determined by individual states.	All uninsured children and adults, regardless of legal status.	All persons (children and adults) enrolled in public and private health care plans.	All children and adults.

continued

TABLE 6-1 Continued

Features	1. VFC (Current System)	2. Expanded VFC	3. Universal Federal Purchase
Who purchases vaccines?	CDC purchases and distributes VFC vaccines.	CDC purchases and distributes VFC vaccines.	CDC purchases and distributes all vaccines for both public and private health care sectors.
Who pays for it?	*Public sector*: Federal government and some states purchase vaccines; administration fees are paid by Medicaid, SCHIP, and state budgets.	*Public sector*: Same as VFC.	*Public sector*: Same as VFC.
	Private sector: Insurers have discretion as to level of coverage for vaccines and administration fees.	*Private sector*: Same as VFC.	*Private sector*: Same as VFC.

4. Federal Block Grant	5. Public Vouchers	6. Insurance Mandate	7. Funded Mandate
State-determined.	Private providers or their insurance plans purchase vaccines. States purchase vaccines on behalf of public clinics.	CDC continues to purchase public-sector vaccines. Providers and insurers purchase vaccines for their enrollees and patients.	Providers purchase all vaccines except for bulk purchases by large insurers seeking discount prices. Insurers (public and private) reimburse providers, and are themselves reimbursed by federal vaccine payments.
Public sector: States purchase vaccines as needed with federal funds, supplemented by discretionary state funding.	*Public sector*: Federal government reimburses providers for cost of vaccine; possibly partial contribution by the states.	*Public sector*: Public health care finance programs (e.g., Medicaid, SCHIP) cover vaccine costs, supplemented by state funding.	*Public sector*: Health care providers, reimbursed by health plans or federal vouchers.
Private sector: Vaccine costs and related fees paid at the discretion of the state.	*Private sector*: Insurers have discretion as to level of coverage for vaccines and fees.	*Private sector*: insurers are required to pay for vaccines and administration fees.	*Private sector*: Health care providers, reimbursed by health plans or federal vouchers.

continued

TABLE 6-1 Continued

Features	1. VFC (Current System)	2. Expanded VFC	3. Universal Federal Purchase
Pros	Federal entitlement assures coverage of eligible populations in most cases. 10-year history associated with rises in vaccine coverage levels. Maintains vaccine delivery in medical home.	Same as VFC. Targets the most critical coverage gaps: underinsured children and uninsured and underinsured high-risk adults. Reduces referrals to the public sector.	Eliminates eligibility questions for all patients and providers. Reduces referrals to the public sector. Eliminates crowd-out.

4. Federal Block Grant	5. Public Vouchers	6. Insurance Mandate	7. Funded Mandate
Allows each state to select the financing approach best suited to its needs.	Eligibility determined at point of issuing voucher, not at point of service.	Targets the most critical coverage gap—underinsured.	Improves incentives for the development of new vaccines.
Enables experimentation to determine optimal mixes of tactics (e.g., vaccine purchases, targeted programs, fees, registries, education, cost sharing).	Reduces provider burden in meeting the needs of the uninsured. Eliminates eligibility problems associated with government purchase of vaccines.	Facilitates state and federal budget planning by stabilizing the population receiving private-sector vaccines. Reduces referrals to public sector clinics.	Eliminates government purchasing of vaccines. Eliminates provider burden in determining eligibility—everyone is covered.
Fosters efficiency by focusing on outcomes.	Reduces referrals to the public sector.	Reduces provider burden in determining eligibility.	Maintains existing community insurer–provider relationships in immunization.
Creates multifaceted market for vaccine purchases; encourages producers to compete in wide range of market configurations.		Eliminates crowd-out. Reduces public market share, enabling the producers to compete in larger private market.	Administration fee is assured.
			Protects consumers from high vaccine costs.
			Facilitates rapid uptake of new vaccines by removing government purchasing delays and health plan reimbursement uncertainties.
			Producers compete in multiple markets.

continued

TABLE 6-1 Continued

Features	1. VFC (Current System)	2. Expanded VFC	3. Universal Federal Purchase
Cons	Strict eligibility requirements create gaps in safety net coverage.	Encourages private insurers to drop immunization coverage (crowd-out).	No private-sector benchmark for pricing.
	Encourages private insurers to drop immunization coverage (crowd-out).	Expands public-sector market share of vaccines, discouraging vaccine industry participation and R&D.	Government is sole customer in vaccine market.
	Fragmented financing system fosters missed opportunities and provider burden.		Supply problems may occur as vaccine producers choose to exit the market or limit production.
	Government purchasing is inefficient; lack of pricing rationale and contracting delays discourage vaccine industry participation and R&D.	Continues fragmented vaccine coverage (creates provider burden).	
		Continues problems associated with of government purchase—pricing uncertainty and contract delays.	

Disadvantages

The two principal disadvantages of the current VFC system are its reliance on government purchase of vaccines and its fragmentation of vaccine financing. As noted earlier, government purchase, which is growing as a share of the total vaccine market, tends to discourage industry invest-

4. Federal Block Grant	5. Public Vouchers	6. Insurance Mandate	7. Funded Mandate
States under fiscal and political pressure may divert funds from immunization programs.	A new federal role and information system investments are required to develop and administer voucher and billing systems.	Cost will be passed to the employer and consumer in the form of higher premiums.	A new federal role and information system investments are required to develop and administer voucher and billing systems.
States may have limited controls with respect to private insurers, such as ERISA.	A substantial burden is involved in locating and tracking changes in eligibility.	Requires monitoring, oversight, and enforcement at both federal and state levels.	A substantial burden is involved in locating and tracking changes in eligibility.
Federal government has limited ability to intervene if ineffective.	Providers may dislike delays in reimbursement associated with vouchers.	Reduces the federal share of the market, possibly reducing federal negotiating leverage.	Providers may dislike delays in reimbursement associated with vouchers.
Requires benchmarks for determining grant awards and performance measures.	Pricing the vouchers requires calculation of the social benefit of vaccines.		Pricing the vouchers and reimbursement plan requires calculation of the social benefit of vaccines.
History of Section 317 funding suggests that many smaller states cannot negotiate reasonable prices with vaccine suppliers.			Requires monitoring, oversight, and enforcement at both federal and state levels.

ment in production capacity and new vaccine R&D. The government price negotiation process itself leads to delays, inefficiencies, and uncertainty about reimbursement among clinicians.

The eligibility limitations of VFC increase the burden on clinicians for eligibility determination; create funding inequities between entitlement and discretionary funding streams (e.g., VFC, Section 317, and state general funds); and fragment the financing and delivery of services, resulting in missed opportunities, scattered records, and fewer children immunized than would otherwise be the case. Moreover, VFC does nothing to help high-risk adults who are either uninsured or underinsured. The separation of vaccine purchases and fees further fragments funding, and results in referrals even of covered children to public-sector clinics. Finally, the VFC financing structure encourages the erosion ("crowd-out") of private coverage because of the existence of public financing.

Alternative 2: Expanded VFC

Description/Design Options

This approach maintains the central features of the current system, and does not change the structure of the VFC program, but expands VFC to include immunization of underinsured children within their medical home. As a result, children who previously could obtain free vaccines only in FQHCs—an estimated 2.7 million children nationwide—would be able to receive vaccines in their medical home. This approach also expands VFC to cover adults who are either under- or uninsured and who are at high risk as defined by CDC.

Advantages

The advantages of the expanded VFC alternative are that it maintains VFC, a time-tested and well-funded program, while making improvements to strengthen coverage. The expanded coverage targets the two most critical coverage gaps: underinsured children and high-risk adults (both uninsured and underinsured). Implementing this alternative would somewhat, but not totally, alleviate eligibility problems that result in missed opportunities and reduce the number of referrals by private providers to the public sector. Among options for changing the current system, this approach would also be the easiest to implement.

Disadvantages

The principal disadvantage associated with the expanded VFC approach is that it maintains and even expands the government's role in purchasing vaccines, potentially discouraging industry investment in production capacity and the development of new vaccines.

Furthermore, while the expansion of coverage would reduce fragmentation, it would not eliminate it; and the burden of eligibility determination on clinicians would remain unaddressed. Crowd-out would be exacerbated, and the separation of vaccine purchases and fees would continue to encourage referrals even of covered children to public-sector clinics. Disparities between entitlement and discretionary program would continue if some states chose to supplement VFC categories with state-purchased vaccines.

The public costs of expanding coverage to include the 3.5 million underinsured children aged 0–5 would be substantial. A national entitlement program is obligated to meet funding levels once eligibility has been established. Hence, the VFC budget grows to meet demand. CDC's fiscal year 2000 budget for immunization was $1.6 billion. This figure includes $990 million for the VFC program and an additional $250 million for Section 317 vaccine purchases (the remaining portion consists of discretionary funds to support state immunization programs).

Immunization would increase among families that could not or would not pay the extra (uncovered) charge for obtaining the vaccine from their private practitioner and who did not have access to a public health clinic for free treatment. How large is this group? Freed et al. (1999) studied the effects of a new universal purchase vaccine program in North Carolina on immunization rates by insurance status. This program provided coverage to the underinsured in much the same way as would the payment plan proposed here. Freed found that the percentage of children who were up to date in immunizations did increase among both those with periods of underinsurance and those with partial coverage (from 80 percent to 86.5 percent for the former and from 85.3 percent to 90.9 percent for the latter, measured at the 24-month point), although his study probably understates the effect since his "preprogram" data were actually collected shortly after the program had begun. There was also some decline in the percentage receiving immunizations at public health clinics, although a significant proportion continued to use the latter facilities.[5] That is not surprising since private physicians would still charge for the visit, even if the vaccine were provided free of charge.

Freed et al. (1999) suggest that increased immunization rates can occur when health professionals and public officials make a big effort to move children into private care. Despite some success, however, it appears that coverage alone does not guarantee these outcomes. It is possible that other factors, such as parents' education, can help explain much

---

[5]Following implementation of the program, the uninsured continued to have the highest usage of public health clinics for vaccinations (52 percent). Public health usage was 35 percent for those with private insurance but partial well-child coverage, 35 percent for those with Medicaid, 43 percent for the underinsured (private insurance, no well-child coverage), and 14 percent for those with private health insurance and full coverage for well-child care.

of the differentially lower rates of vaccination and higher rates of use of public health clinics among subgroups with different types of coverage.

Alternative 3: Universal Federal Purchase

Description/Design Options

Under this approach, the federal government purchases all routinely recommended childhood vaccines. These vaccines are distributed by the states through existing VFC mechanisms. All children are vaccinated with publicly acquired vaccines, regardless of their health insurance status or care setting. All children from birth through 18 years of age are covered under this approach; adult vaccines could be covered as well.

CDC would continue negotiate a contract price for each vaccine. But in contrast to the current method, CDC would calculate a value for the societal benefit of each vaccine and set a price as some percentage of that amount. Provider administration fees could be mandated as an option, and states could use Section 317 funds to support payment of those fees.

Advantages

This approach has many advantages. All children would be covered under all circumstances. Eligibility determination would be eliminated, and providers would no longer have to maintain multiple stocks of vaccines. No children would have to be referred from private to public clinics because of ineligibility to receive the vaccine on hand. Children could remain in their medical homes for immunization services. Because states would be expanding their childhood vaccine distribution system, the contact between public health departments and private providers could be enhanced, likely promoting improvements in immunization-related activities, such as participation in population-based immunization registries.

A price based on societal benefit might be higher than a price based on such factors as the market power of the purchaser. However, it would express the maximum amount that society would be willing to pay for the vaccine, and provide a more adequate incentive for R&D and assure a continuous supply of those vaccines that are developed and marketed.

Disadvantages

The principal disadvantage of this approach is the continuation and expansion of the government purchase system. If government were to utilize its additional monopsony power to reduce prices, such action could lead to further shortages, exacerbate market exit, and choke off R&D. Even if the proposed pricing model yielded higher prices, the risk of future price reductions could make investment in R&D appear less attractive. The industry's uncertainty about future pricing is one of the key issues associated with any government-funded program. If the private market for vaccines were virtually eliminated, there would be no theoretical basis for determining appropriate prices; and industry would be at risk for a change in government procurement policy, for example, as part of a federal-deficit reduction initiative.

The public costs of this alternative would be quite substantial—possibly doubling the federal government's vaccine budget, even at current prices. Congress has consistently rejected universal, single-payor programs, although a single-payor approach for vaccines may be more palatable in this case given that these services have strong public-good properties and are a small component of overall health spending. Vaccine manufacturers are also likely to oppose a universal purchase proposal. Although manufacturers are used to universal government purchase programs through their western European operations, they rely on the U.S. market as a source of profits to support R&D.

Only indirect evidence exists in support of this approach. For example, many other countries that have universal government acquisition of vaccines have higher vaccination levels than those of the United States. In those states that have implemented their own versions of universal purchase arrangements, however, significantly higher childhood immunization rates have not been achieved as compared with states that rely exclusively on the current less-than-universal federal government purchase programs.[6]

Other concerns include the erosion of long-standing community and health plan relationships that have evolved as a result of the mixed public–private system; the continued separation of vaccine purchases and fees; and the potential windfall to health plans, which might not adjust premiums immediately despite the elimination of vaccine costs.

Alternative 4: Federal Block Grant

Description/Design Options

Under this approach, states receive annual grants for immunization from the federal government. The government calculates the grant using

---

[6]Between 1997 and 2001, average immunization rates for the 3:4:1:3 series increased as follows: 74.1–77.3 percent in VFC-only states, 74.2–77.8 percent in enhanced-VFC states, 78.7–80.9 percent in limited universal purchase states, and 78.0–78.1 percent in universal purchase states (CDC, 2002a; CDC, 1998; calculations by the committee).

a formula based on current VFC funding and other variables. States must meet certain immunization targets to avoid penalties, including loss of the grant. The states have broad discretion in how they allocate the funds among the various immunization-related activities, such as purchasing vaccines, investing in infrastructure, paying administrative fees, conducting targeted immunizations, enhancing registries, and providing education and outreach services. States also determine eligibility for public programs.

Advantages

This approach has two principal advantages. First, it would encourage innovation by allowing states to try different approaches and combinations of inputs (e.g., vaccines, infrastructure, education) to optimize their program. Second, this approach would allow programs to be customized to the particular needs and environment of each state, which vary considerably. The focus on outcomes would reinforce the opportunities for experimentation.

This approach would also create a decentralized, nonfederal market for the purchase of vaccines, which would enable vaccine companies to compete across states and across a range of product and service configurations. The impact on prices cannot be predicted: the loss of federal monopsony power would result in increased prices, all else being equal; but this might be balanced by the development of large purchasing consortia and the higher degree of price sensitivity of states.

Disadvantages

The principal concern with regard to block grants in general—whether maternal and child health, education, or other social service programs—is the possibility that states would find ways to divert the funds to other purposes, especially when faced with pressure to reduce their total budgets. Clearly designated outcomes and performance measures could help prevent such diversion of funds, but enforcement might be difficult and highly political. Moreover, the level of block grant funding, being discretionary, could be threatened from year to year and would be subject to jockeying for advantage among the states. Block grant formulas are widely perceived as being notoriously difficult to make truly equitable. For example, states could find a wide range of vaccine prices based on their size and negotiating clout, resulting in an inequitable cost burden across states and exacerbating disparities in immunization rates.

In addition, despite regional differences, infectious disease control may be better suited to management by regional or national authorities.

Immunization's public-good characteristics are national in scope—epidemics do not respect state borders—and states could become "free-riders," particularly in times of fiscal stress. The elimination of programmatic funding through federal agencies could impair tracking and consistent enforcement, adversely impact federal–state collaboration, and make it difficult for the federal government to provide guidance or to intervene should a state program fail to meet minimum targets. By adopting very different approaches, states could lose the ability to draw useful comparisons or to coordinate effectively in case of regional outbreaks.

Alternative 5: Public Vouchers for Vaccine Purchase

Description/Design Options

As in alternative 4, the voucher approach devolves vaccine purchasing from the government to insurers, states, and providers. Under this approach, a voucher is given to each eligible person (including both children and high-risk adults) to cover some percentage of the cost of each vaccine and the associated provider fee. The person can then spend the voucher at any provider of his or her choice. In their basic design, these vouchers are similar to food stamps. The amount of the voucher is set in advance and may cover all or part of the vaccine purchase price. Vaccines can be purchased directly by providers or purchased by states, clinics, hospitals, insurers, or other entities and supplied to providers. If the voucher is set at an amount below the total of the purchase price and administration fee, the provider can bill the patient for the difference. The voucher as envisioned by the committee covers all uninsured children and adults.

The committee considered many specific design alternatives:

- Providing universal coverage versus means testing the voucher.
- Setting the voucher amount to cover the full cost of vaccines or less than the full cost.
- If less than the full cost, means testing the cost sharing, or not.
- Using an electronic card system, paper vouchers, or simply physician billing for each vaccine administered.

There are trade-offs involved in all of these approaches. For example, covering all children would be expensive, but would be the easiest approach to administer. Means testing the voucher, on the other hand, would require a significant administrative apparatus to enroll children in the voucher program, establish eligibility, and monitor and pay claims. Preserving some consumer responsibility through the use of cost sharing, however, would reward families for seeking out low-cost providers, thereby helping to contain the costs of the system.

For those with insurance, the eligible person would receive a voucher or credit equal to the annual actuarial value of vaccinations provided; this credit could be used to cover any direct premium or to offset lower wages associated with employer-provided insurance or signed over to the employer or union that makes the payment for the family's insurance. The purpose of this provision is to avoid an incentive to employers and eligible employees to drop coverage in order to be eligible for a voucher (i.e., to avoid "crowd-out"), to permit administrative cost economies derived from having a single insurer administer all types of medical care for employment-group members at all income levels, and to achieve equitable treatment of those who obtain insurance coverage that substitutes for direct vouchers. If the administrative cost of instituting insurance vouchers for recommended immunizations were high in absolute terms and relative to the value of the voucher, the direct payment mechanism might be extended to those currently having coverage as well. Crowd-out would then be expected but would be tolerated in the interest of administrative simplicity.

Advantages

A principal advantage of the voucher approach is that eligibility is determined at the time the voucher is issued, not at the point of service, thus relieving providers of this onerous and difficult administrative task. Vouchers would also eliminate the clinician's uncertainty about eventual reimbursement (aside from government reimbursement delays). Since providers would themselves decide where and how to purchase vaccines, there would be no need to segregate vaccine supplies for different categories of patients. The voucher approach would probably result in fewer lost opportunities for vaccination by reducing referrals away from the patient's medical home.

The voucher approach would also promote efficiency by putting purchasing power directly in the hands of the needy population, giving the recipient free choice of a provider. The federal government would no longer purchase vaccines or negotiate vaccine prices, except perhaps for vaccines with only a single seller. State governments could elect to purchase vaccine supplies for resale to physicians in the state, especially if the state believed it could negotiate a favorable price.

The electronic voucher card option would facilitate the development of a central registry. Having such a registry would assist in surveillance, reduce missed opportunities, and prevent duplicate vaccinations that can occur when charts are not available at the point of service.

There is also considerable flexibility in the way a voucher system can be designed, and its payment structure can be manipulated easily from a central point. For example, to provide extra incentives for vaccination in special circumstances, such as outbreak control or difficult-to-reach categories of children, the value of the voucher could be set higher than the outlay cost; for example, a family in a rural area could receive an additional payment to reflect greater travel costs.

Vaccine companies would likely support a program that reduced federal purchasing and enabled them to compete. There has also been experience with successful government voucher programs—such as food stamps and college loans through the GI bill and other federal programs—that could provide guidance in setting up a vaccine voucher system.

Disadvantages

The principal disadvantage of the voucher approach is its administrative complexity and cost of implementation, particularly with regard to investments in information technology and the workforce required to establish eligibility for the vouchers. Tying the program to existing programs, such as Medicaid, would simplify its implementation. Also, some of these problems would be considerably reduced with a universal voucher.

A voucher system would be a new program, with attendant costs of set-up and education. Many design details would have to be addressed, including eligibility; enrollment systems; and computer linkages for cards, doctors' offices, and reimbursement centers. Particularly challenging would be determining a voucher price that would balance providing sufficient return on investment to the vaccine industry to encourage continued supply and investment in R&D; protecting taxpayers from exorbitant increases in vaccine prices; and avoiding significant increases in patient cost sharing, which can present a barrier to immunization.

The administrative disadvantages of the voucher system could be minimized, however, through alternative approaches. A magnetic card or paper voucher, like a food stamp, would give the consumer full control of the purchase decision and the ability to shop for the best quality and price. At the same time, it would ensure that the provider would accept the voucher by making it simple to use and redeem. The provider would not need to assess eligibility—possession of the voucher would be sufficient.

An essential difference exists, however, between food stamps and vaccines. Because medical providers have established procedures for submitting claims for services rendered, they could easily integrate a paper voucher into their billing system. Thus, a physical voucher might not be necessary in the case of vaccines. For example, providers could immunize a patient and submit a bill to the federal vaccine authority, which would reimburse the provider for all vaccine claims on a regular basis, allocating the payment to the appropriate program based on the patient's eligibility. While there are certain advantages to the paper or electronic card version of the voucher approach, its administrative complexity would be enormous.

A substantial disadvantage of a voucher system that excluded adults not at high risk is that many adults with high-risk indications would go unrecognized and, as a consequence, would remain unvaccinated. The voucher approach would require that high-risk adults be identified as such in advance for the purpose of obtaining the voucher, so that the voucher would be available when needed. But physicians could have a difficult time identifying patients with high-risk indications for immunization.

Alternative 6: Insurance Mandate

Description/Design Options

This approach requires that all insurers, both public and private, provide coverage to all enrollees, with limits on the deductibles, copayments, and coinsurance they can require. While 28 states have already imposed mandates on state-regulated insurers, this approach involves a federal requirement that applies to both state- and federally-regulated insurers and employer plans (AAP, 2003). Insurers would be required to report on vaccine coverage and cost sharing to the government. The mandate would apply to any vaccine that has low insurance coverage rates (i.e., more than 5 percent of the target population remains uninsured for the vaccine) 5 years after the introduction of the vaccine or after the initiation of the program.

This approach is contingent on a redesign of the ACIP recommendation process. ACIP's decisions have enormous private- and public-sector financial implications. Given the rising costs of vaccines, combined with the less-favorable cost–benefit profiles of some current and pipeline vaccines, ACIP has a responsibility to make economic considerations central to its recommendation function. Under this approach, ACIP would establish multiple tiers for vaccine recommendations. One tier would include vaccines with strong spillover effects because of the highly infectious nature of the diseases they prevent. The mandate would apply principally to these vaccines. The committee's proposed approach with respect to ACIP is described fully in Chapter 7.

Advantages

The mandate approach targets the most important coverage gaps—underinsured children and high-risk adults (both underinsured and uninsured). In addition, by eliminating crowd-out and reducing referrals from private to public providers, the approach would add stability to the immunization system and enhance the ability of federal and state governments to estimate needs and plan accordingly. Reduced referrals would result in less fragmentation of care and thus fewer missed opportunities and duplicate immunizations. The mandate approach would also alleviate the provider burden by greatly reducing the problem of eligibility determination.

The emphasis on tier-one vaccines would foster a more stable and predictable growth in vaccine costs over time and send clear signals to the industry about the societal priorities for vaccine development. The reduced public market share would appeal to producers because it would enable them to compete in a larger private market.

Disadvantages

The principal disadvantage of an insurance mandate is that the costs of increased coverage are likely to be passed on to either consumers, in the form of higher copayments and deductibles, or their employers, in the form of higher premiums. Although vaccines represent a relatively small share of insurer costs, that share is expected to increase substantially with the addition of new vaccines to the schedule. Mandating coverage could drive companies to drop coverage altogether, particularly in a weak economy, thereby increasing the number of uninsured. Moreover, while the burden on providers for determining eligibility would be alleviated by the elimination of the distinction between those who are fully insured and those who are underinsured within the insured population, determination of eligibility within public programs would remain burdensome.

Furthermore, while the mandate would technically eliminate insurance crowd-out, referrals of privately insured patients to the public sector for immunizations could increase nonetheless. Past experience with both VFC maintenance-of-effort laws and state mandates suggests that substantial investments in regulatory infrastructure could be required to ensure compliance with the mandate and to control the rate of referrals from the private to the public sector.

The government's market share in vaccine purchases would decrease under this alternative, reducing the monopsony power of the government and its ability to negotiate steep discounts. The committee views this lifting of pressure on prices positively in terms of investment in production capacity and R&D; however, it could have adverse short-term impacts on states, programs, and providers.

Alternative 7: Funded Mandate

Description/Design Options

The funded mandate alternative combines elements of the voucher approach and the insurance mandate. The mandate requires that both public and private insurers provide coverage for all insured children, all adults over age 65, and certain designated populations, such as adults aged 18–64 who are at particular risk for the consequences of vaccine-preventable disease because of certain health disorders. The insurers' costs of providing this mandated coverage are reimbursed in full by the federal government. Insurers purchase vaccines directly and receive reimbursement at the subsidy rate. Health plans are required to reimburse their providers the full replacement cost of the vaccine up to the subsidy amount, plus the full administration fee. If the health plan or provider can obtain vaccines at a price below the federal subsidy amount, they can keep the difference. Patients who are uninsured receive a voucher for immunization as described under alternative 5 above.

The amount of the federal subsidy is some percentage of a vaccine's calculated social benefit, announced in advance of the release of the vaccine to stimulate the pace of development. A method for determining a price in advance based on the calculated societal benefit is described by McGuire (2003) (see Box 6-1). Societal benefit, as defined by the committee, is a measure of the total benefits provided by a vaccine, including both private benefits to those who receive the vaccine and public benefits that accrue to the rest of society. These benefits include direct medical costs saved because the disease was prevented, as well as such benefits as increased length of life and improved quality of life. Under this alternative, prices of current vaccines are determined based on some combination of calculated social benefit and past prices.

Advantages

This approach shares many of the advantages of the voucher and mandate alternatives. It would increase incentives for the development of new vaccines by providing manufacturers with assurance of adequate pricing and returns. Furthermore, the assurance of a price subsidy based on societal benefit would steer innovation toward the most socially beneficial vaccines. An additional advantage of this approach to setting a price subsidy is that it would require no reference to industry cost data.

Funding the insurance mandate would maintain the insurer's role in immunization, avoid disruption of existing infrastructure, preserve established community networks, and prevent referrals from physicians to public-sector providers. It would create market mechanisms by allowing insurers and physicians to keep savings they might obtain, and thereby stimulate efficiency and competition among vaccine producers, who would enjoy competition in multiple markets—physicians, institutions, states, and purchasing cooperatives. This approach would eliminate government purchasing and the concomitant delays and uncertainties in reimbursement.

A key difference between the subsidy approach and a universal purchase approach is in the way prices are determined. Currently, the price of a vaccine is determined in two ways. In the private sector, it is based on "what the market will bear." In the public sector, it is based on a negotiation between CDC and the manufacturers, usually resulting in a substantial discount. To stimulate additional investment in R&D, each of the alternative approaches considered by the committee seeks to increase the rate of return on vaccine products within reasonable limits. The approaches pursue this goal in different ways. Under a universal purchase approach (alternative 3), the government would purchase all vaccines. It could raise prices to stimulate investment, or it could drop prices if they were too high. The fact is, however, that government would have no basis for raising or lowering prices because there would no longer be any market reference price for comparison. Absent such a benchmark, pricing would become a political process, which would create uncertainty regarding future prices and likely reduce industry investment in R&D.

The case of a genetically engineered protein that helps reduce anemia in dialysis patients is instructive with regard to the potential for politicization of pricing. This product is covered under Medicare for all individuals (including those under age 65). There is some evidence that the initial price of the new product provided a very high return on R&D to the manufacturer, as well as a high benefit–cost value for society. Its initial price was negotiated between the Health Care Financing Administration (HCFA) and the manufacturer and subsequently codified in legislative amendments (with discretion on the part of HCFA to adjust prices for inflation). Subsequently, the product was the subject of several favorable benefit–cost studies by economists. But the Clinton Administration and several congressmen thought that expenditures exceeded budgets, and congressional action decreased the price. Similar approaches to vaccines that reflected arbitrary government pricing would be devastating to vaccine R&D.

Under a subsidy approach, individual providers or health insurance plans would purchase vaccines and would then be reimbursed by gov-

BOX 6-1
Setting Prices for New Vaccines in Advance

The economic return to vaccine development appears to be low. The number of firms producing vaccines for the United States has declined (Rappouli et al., 2002), and research and development (R&D) on new vaccines appears not to be pursued as aggressively as is warranted by the social return involved. The majority of R&D effort is apparently directed toward diseases for which there is already a vaccine, rather than the discovery of new vaccines (Finkelstein, 2003). Thus pricing policies are not directing industry R&D to solve problems involving the highest social return. Given the strong public-good properties of vaccines (see Box 2-1 in Chapter 2), a case can be made for public intervention to increase the returns to vaccine R&D (Kremer, 2000a).

Anticipated profits drive R&D in both pharmaceuticals and vaccines (Finklestein, 2003; Grabowski and Vernon, 2000; Scherer, 2001). The price for a vaccine rewards the innovator firm, which spurs investment in future vaccine development. But a high price also reduces the net benefit to consumers of current vaccines.

The trade-off between incentives to develop new vaccines and short-term fairness and efficiency is addressed by McGuire (2003).[1] McGuire considers how to set a price for a vaccine not yet developed that balances these two goals. This price would be high enough to create a desirable level of R&D, but low enough to assure substantial public benefit once a product has been developed. It should be noted that, while McGuire's approach informed the committee's deliberations, the committee's approach differs in important ways.

The Model

To find a price that balances increased innovation and short-term efficiency, McGuire proposes a pricing model based on economic theory (Laffont, 1994).[2]

First he determines the efficient level of spending on R&D that maximizes the expected net benefits accruing from the activity. The efficient level of investment in R&D is the x that maximizes expression (a).

Expected net benefit = $q(x)[b - c] - x$ (a)

where

---

[1]Thomas McGuire's paper *Setting Prices for New Vaccines (In Advance)*, is available from IOM and will be published in the *International Journal of Health Care Finance and Economics* (forthcoming).

[2]There are interesting parallels to defense contracting issues (Rogerson, 1994).

b is the average per-person benefit of eliminating the disease,
x is the per–person expenditure on R&D,
q(x) is the probability of successful discovery of a vaccine, and
c is the marginal production cost.

Second, McGuire defines the level of R&D that maximizes the expected profits of the producer:

$$\text{Expected profits} = q(x)[p - c] - x \tag{b}$$

where

p is the price of the vaccine.

The firm's choice of *x* to maximize profits would be identical to the social objective of choosing *x* to maximize net social benefit if *price = average benefit*. Therefore, the efficient price for a vaccine is equal to the average benefit from the vaccine. But by setting *price = average benefit*, all of this expected net benefit appears as profits, and none as consumer benefit. If all net social benefits are transferred to the supplier, the consumer is no better off with the vaccine than without.

Third, the optimal price from the consumer's point of view is determined. This price is represented by *expected consumer surplus*, which is the difference between the benefits and price of the vaccine, times the likelihood of the vaccine being discovered (expression (c)). The trade-off involved in setting a price is evident in this expression. To increase consumer surplus *[b – p]*, price must be lowered. But a lower price will lead to lower *x*, and therefore a reduced chance that the vaccine will be available.

$$\text{Consumer surplus} = q(x)[b - p] \tag{c}$$

The problem is to find the price that maximizes consumer surplus subject to maximization of firm profits. The optimal price is governed by how *q(x)*, the likely success of research, depends on the level of investment.

Putting the Model into Practice

The usual approach to cost–benefit assessment in health policy is to consider the welfare of buyers only, ignoring profits as part of social benefits. By including profits, McGuire's approach balances society's long-term and short-term goals. But in addition to reliable estimates of the social benefits of a vaccine, this approach requires an estimate of production costs and knowledge of the relationship between investment in R&D and likely success (the "research production function").

continued

BOX 6-1 Continued

A recent Institute of Medicine (IOM) report provides a starting point for considering whether benefits can be operationalized (IOM, 2000b). Using a common analytical framework, an IOM panel calculated costs and benefits of 26 vaccines in the R&D pipeline. For inputs, McGuire used IOM's calculations of vaccine benefits, estimated production costs, and derived a standard research production function using economic theory.

McGuire calculated two optimal prices for each vaccine (see the table below). The first gives 80 percent of the surplus to consumers, and the second divides the surplus 50/50. Social efficiency (i.e., total surplus) increases as the share given to consumers declines. (Prices shown are per person vaccinated, not per dose.) For purposes of comparison, at current CDC contract prices, invasive pneumococcal and varicella vaccines cost about $184 and $41 per person, respectively (including all doses).

Setting a high price (e.g., $200 for a vaccine against cytomegalovirus) would accelerate the development of a vaccine with large social benefits. Prices could also be chosen for other vaccines against diseases, perhaps in the range of 50–80 percent benefit to consumers. Private industry could then make decisions about the pursuit of vaccines against these diseases on the basis of their own technical knowledge of the likelihood of finding a vaccine, as well as the social value of the vaccine itself.

Sensitivity analysis shows that a price set too low reduces consumer surplus, profits, and social welfare. Setting a price too high, however, reduces consumer surplus but increases profits and social welfare. The analysis suggests that to deal with the considerable uncertainty associated with estimating social benefit, the best strategy is to err on the high side.

McGuire's formal model requires that subsidy rates reflect the likelihood of success of new vaccine efforts. If one uses just realized benefits on successful R&D, firms will be paid only a fraction of the amount required for them to take the risk of trying yet-unproven ideas. It is unclear how an adjustment for this could be incorporated or how one might prevent abuse of the system or underprovision.

The notion of setting a price in advance is not entirely novel. The commitment and general policy proposed here are similar to the Countermeasure Purchase Fund proposed by Senator Lieberman in S1764 (December 4, 2001), "Research to Develop Vaccine and Medicines to Treat Victims of Bio-Terrorism Attacks." Specifically, "This legislation provides that a company that successfully develops a countermeasure—through FDA approval—is eligible to sell the product to the Federal government at a pre-established price and in a pre-determined amount."

A major uncertainty for industry would be eliminated by prices set in advance. If the public sector committed to a price, more investment would follow because of expected revenue and because of the reduction in risk.

Illustrative Results of Pricing Model				
Analysis Steps and Assumptions	S. pneumoniae	Group B Streptococcus (GBS)	Chlamydia	Cyto-megalo-virus
IOM cost-effectiveness estimates Present value of annualized health costs ($ mil)	$1,600	$630	$850	$4,000
Present value of annualized QALYs	265,000	37,400	525,000	70,000
Calculations Cost savings per person	$201	$79	$107	$503
Value of QALY per person	$50	$7	$99	$13
Total benefits per person	$251	$86	$206	$516
Pricing 80% benefit to consumer surplus	$58	$25	$49	$111
50% benefit to consumer surplus	$130	$48	$108	$263
Assumptions QALY value:	$50,000			
U.S. population:	265 million			
Discount rate:	3.0%			
Production cost per dose: $10				

NOTE: QALY = quality-adjusted life year.

ernment payments at a certain percentage of their cost. In many cases, the price of the vaccine would shift to the subsidy amount, which would be set at a level that would encourage manufacturers to invest in R&D. There could be differences, however, between the subsidy amount and the price paid. Manufacturers could charge more than the subsidy, although doing so would remove the vaccine from the mandate. Manufactures could also charge lower prices in response to the negotiating leverage of large purchasers or buying cooperatives. But even if prices stayed at the subsidy level, manufacturers would still be able to compete on the basis of quality, service, and product enhancements. Thus, while the subsidy might equal the market price in many cases, it would preserve some aspects of the market. This alternative would also provide a formula-based method for setting the subsidy that would be less subject to political manipulation than pure government purchasing. While no strong evidentiary base clearly establishes the relative superiority of different approaches to setting such a subsidy, a government purchase approach would be untenable to manufacturers.

Disadvantages

By combining features of the voucher and insurance mandate alternatives, this strategy some of the disadvantages of each. The most serious of these is the complexity of having two separate administrative and regulatory functions—one to administer the voucher and one to monitor and enforce the mandate.

This approach could also be expected to increase federal expenditures for vaccines at least as much as and probably substantially more than any of the other alternatives. Higher costs would result from both expanded public coverage and higher prices. One of the key practical issues would be how to determine a subsidy amount that would encourage vaccine development without allowing expenditures to increase more than necessary. While this approach would preserve a private market for vaccines, using a subsidy based on the calculated societal benefit of a vaccine could stimulate prices to increase substantially to subsidy levels. As McGuire (2003) explains, if a subsidy formula allows prices to rise to the level of the calculated societal benefit, no benefit will remain for the consumer. The calculation of societal benefits and of subsidy amounts based on those benefits presents a variety of technical challenges and could require politically difficult legislative decisions regarding key assumptions used in the calculations.

Finally, implementation of this alternative would require substantial amendments to established law in numerous areas (e.g., Employee Retirement Income Security Act, Public Health Act, Medicare, Medicaid,

SCHIP). A comprehensive legislative strategy would be necessary to reduce the risk of an incremental and uneven approach.

WEIGHING THE ALTERNATIVES

Each strategy outlined above has certain advantages and disadvantages in addressing the two key objectives addressed by the committee: (1) assuring access to recommended vaccines and (2) sustaining the availability of vaccines in the future. The decision process used by the committee in selecting among these alternatives was an exercise in identifying and making difficult trade-offs that often involved direct conflicts between these objectives. For example, two of the approaches—expanding the eligibility categories for VFC and moving to a universal purchase system—address primarily the access objective by eliminating underinsurance and reducing incentives for providers to refer patients away from their routine source of care for immunizations. But both approaches expand government involvement in the purchase of vaccines, and thus potentially undermine investment in production capacity and the development of new vaccines by the vaccine industry. In contrast, the block grant approach emphasizes the importance of a decentralized, pluralistic market that would likely encourage competition and investment in the vaccine industry. But the block grant approach could be detrimental to access by fragmenting eligibility and funding streams, and creating multiple standards that would limit federal oversight and control in the event of a multi-state outbreak.

Other approaches involve more practical problems. Vouchers, for example, would foster pluralistic markets in which government intervention would be limited to subsidizing the purchase of vaccines. Vouchers would both encourage vaccine industry investment and improve access by relieving clinicians of the burden of checking eligibility requirements for vaccine purchases. But using vouchers as the principal mechanism for financing immunization for children and eligible adults would require the creation of an enormous administrative infrastructure for a relatively small benefit.

The alternatives examined by the committee vary substantially in their complexity in terms of both legislative and implementation requirements. A straightforward expansion of VFC, for example, would be both legislatively simpler and easier to implement than other alternatives. Moreover, an alternative to implementing a new policy immediately is to wait for the results of new research and demonstration projects, and certain aspects of the alternative approaches are more amenable to research and demonstration than others. For example, a demonstration of a voucher system implemented in a few sites would likely reveal much about the system's practicality, acceptance, cost, and effectiveness. Conversely, a demonstration of changes in the federal purchasing system would not succeed because the desired market effects on pricing and industry investment could not be tested in selected locations. Nevertheless, evaluation research would be valuable during the implementation phase of any of these alternatives to monitor its impact and permit midcourse adjustments to fine-tune the policy.

Summary of Recommendations

Recommendation 1: The committee recommends the implementation of a new insurance mandate, combined with a government subsidy and voucher plan, for vaccines recommended by the Advisory Committee on Immunization Practices (ACIP).

Recommendation 2: The Secretary of the Department of Health and Human Services should propose changes in the procedures and membership of ACIP so that its recommendations can associate vaccine coverage decisions with social benefits and costs, including consideration of the impact of the price of a vaccine on recommendations for its use.

Recommendation 3: As part of the implementation of recommendations 1 and 2, the National Vaccine Program Office should convene a series of stakeholder deliberations on the administrative, technical, and legislative issues associated with a shift from vaccine purchase to a vaccine mandate, subsidy, and voucher finance strategy. In addition, the Centers for Disease Control and Prevention (CDC) should sponsor a postimplementation evaluation study (in 5 years, for example). CDC should also initiate a research program aimed at improving the measurement of the societal value of vaccines, addressing methodological challenges, and providing a basis for comparing the impact of different measurement approaches in achieving national immunization goals.

7

Recommendations

The national immunization system, and the Vaccines for Children (VFC) program in particular, has been highly successful to date. But the system has yet to attain national immunization goals for children, and new challenges now threaten the accomplishments that have been made. Policy makers today face daunting challenges related to persistent disparities, missed opportunities in the administration of vaccines, recent vaccine shortages, higher costs of new vaccines, and the growing fragmentation and complexity of public and private financing and delivery of vaccines.

Developing a social policy for vaccine pricing and procurement requires consideration of multiple objectives, each of which sends different signals to the pharmaceutical industry, purchasers, providers, and the public. Different incentive structures influence the trade-offs involved among different purchasing or pricing strategies. To achieve high immunization rates, for example, government agencies frequently strive to reduce financial barriers that inhibit the demand for or administration of vaccines. This goal has led to a pricing policy that seeks to limit public expenditures, in some cases through forceful negotiation of public prices for new vaccine products and through administrative and legislative price caps on certain older vaccines (Miller, 2002). Similarly, public insurers, such as Medicaid and Medicare, have limited the vaccine administration fees paid to physicians and other health care providers.

Assuring access to vaccines is therefore only one objective that shapes vaccine procurement policy. In recent years, several reports have directed attention to the effect of government pricing and purchasing practices on the vaccine market and supply system (GAO, 2002; NVAC, 2003). Some observers have indicated that current government purchasing policies are inadequate because the growing scope of the public-sector market and price controls discourages investments in vaccine development and production capacity (Miller, 2002; Rappuoli et al., 2002).

The challenge now is to develop financial strategies that can achieve multiple objectives rather than perpetuating incremental approaches that satisfy some limited interests at the expense of others. The objectives to be pursued include supplying vaccines to the children and adults who need them, compensating the industries that produce vaccines at rates that reflect the social benefits of vaccines and also encourage the development of new vaccine products, and allowing the government greater discretion in determining the level of investment it is prepared to make in procuring new vaccines compared with other areas of disease prevention and treatment. The committee determined that achieving the dual objectives of assuring high rates of immunization and encouraging innovation requires a rethinking of the current policies and practices by which federal and state agencies recommend, purchase, and administer vaccines. Incremental reforms may help resolve a short-term crisis or strengthen an isolated component of this dynamic and interactive system, but piecemeal approaches will do little to foster a coherent strategy that can align national health policy goals with the desired outcomes. Even the VFC entitlement, which has been credited with achieving substantial gains in immunization rates, is now struggling with budgetary and contracting delays and eligibility requirements that interfere with its ability to provide a reliable and sustainable safety net for a growing number of new and expensive vaccine products.[1] Mandating coverage for vaccines within all insurance plans without providing some mechanism for insurers, employers, and individuals to recover escalating costs could lead to high numbers of uninsured persons; it could also lead some individuals either to pay higher fees (in the form of premiums or deductibles) to obtain coverage or to forego vaccination. Such issues require close attention to the ways in which the immunization burden is shared between the public and private health sectors during periods of escalating health care costs.

In framing its recommendations, the committee focused its analysis on the seven alternative approaches described in Chapter 6. Each ap-

---

[1]A series of improvements in the financing of childhood vaccines announced by President Bush as part of the fiscal year 2004 budget (U.S. Department of Health and Human Services, 2003) occurred after the final meeting of this committee and were not considered during its deliberations. Although these budgetary proposals address some of the committee's concerns, they are short-term solutions that do not resolve key systemic problems addressed by the committee's proposed financing strategy.

proach was considered in terms of its impact on the twin goals outlined earlier in this report: (1) assuring access to current vaccines for all children and adults and (2) assuring the availability of future vaccines by encouraging private investment in the continued production of current vaccines, as well as the development of new vaccine products. In addition, the committee sought to design a strategy that would maintain a reasonable budget for vaccine purchases for children and adults in the public and private health sectors.

RECOMMENDATIONS

Chapter 6 describes the advantages and disadvantages of seven alternative vaccine finance strategies that represent a broad menu of choices for policy makers. Although each approach has advantages and disadvantages, the committee ultimately adopted one of these seven strategies as its principal recommendation, supported by two additional recommendations.

Recommendation 1: The committee recommends the implementation of a new insurance mandate, combined with a government subsidy and voucher plan, for vaccines recommended by the Advisory Committee on Immunization Practices (ACIP).

The proposed plan, referred to as the *vaccine payment system*, consists of five core components that should be considered an integrated strategy for achieving the key objectives of access and availability of vaccines:

• Federal legislation would be required to establish a vaccination coverage mandate for all public and private health plans. This mandate would apply to both state-regulated insurance plans and self-funded employer plans (which are exempt from state regulation under the Employee Retirement Income Security Act [ERISA]), as well as Medicare, Medicaid, the State Children's Health Insurance Program (SCHIP), and government health plans for military personnel and civilian employees. The mandate would provide vaccine benefits for all insured children; adults aged 65 and older; and certain designated populations, such as adults aged 18–64 who have certain health disorders that place them at higher risk for vaccine-preventable disease.
• The federal government would create a new federal subsidy to reimburse public and private health plans and providers for mandated vaccine costs and associated vaccine administration fees.
• The federal government would also create a voucher system for vaccines and vaccine administration fees for designated uninsured populations.

- The insurance mandate, subsidy, and voucher would apply principally to vaccines that have substantial spillover effects as a result of their ability to prevent highly contagious diseases. Vaccines without substantial spillover effects, such as therapeutic vaccines, would be considered for inclusion only in cases of exceptional societal benefit.

- The amount of the subsidy and voucher would be determined both for vaccines currently on the immunization schedule and for vaccines that are not yet available. The subsidy for new vaccines would be based on an estimate of their societal benefit. The subsidy for vaccines already in use would be based on a formula that takes into account both current market price and their calculated societal benefit. The mandate would not apply to vaccines that are priced above the subsidy amount.

Major Features. A government-funded insurance mandate for immunization represents a reformulation of a universal vaccine purchase program and would assure that clinically appropriate immunization services would become a basic and required feature of all public and private health insurance plans. This strategy changes the role of government from one of buying vaccines to one of assuring immunization by providing a fixed subsidy that is adequate to reimburse both vaccine costs and administration fees for public and private insurers and clinicians. As a universal program, the government vaccine subsidy is extended to all persons within the designated populations. As a payment reimbursement program, it sustains the role of government in subsidizing the cost of immunization and enhances incentives for investment in vaccine products, but it reduces the impact of government purchases on the vaccine market relative to other approaches (such as a universal purchase policy).

The prospect of a guaranteed public subsidy for selected vaccines would provide economic incentives that would encourage manufacturers to invest in the clinical trial, licensing, and production processes necessary to move a vaccine product from the early stage of discovery to its use in routine medical care. Reducing the financial uncertainties associated with these processes would stimulate the market and encourage the development of new and effective vaccine products.

At the same time, the federal subsidy for vaccines would not provide a blank check for a new vaccine product. The process of establishing a predetermined subsidy for vaccines not yet marketed would offer incentives for reliable and innovative vaccine product development, while also encouraging efficiency and competition in the production process. Specific features of the recommended strategy are reviewed below, followed by a discussion of its advantages, disadvantages, and implementation issues. Figure 7-1 illustrates the process proposed by the committee.

Mandate Requirements. If vaccines are to continue to be offered within settings for routine medical care, it is essential for all health plans that cover basic health care services to include all vaccines recommended for their enrolled populations. The proposed mandate would extend to populations registered for services through contractual agreements with public health clinics. It would reduce the current administrative burden associated with screening for eligibility and the missed opportunities related to time-consuming referrals of underinsured populations to public health settings—both of which create inefficiencies within the health care system and reduce immunization rates. The proposed mandate would also reduce the variations existing among states that have adopted universal purchase, enhanced VFC, and VFC-only policies.

Because most health plans already cover childhood vaccines, the inclusion of vaccine benefits would not be unduly burdensome for most insurance plans and their purchasers. Nor would the mandate add an extra burden to government health plans such as Medicaid, SCHIP, or Medicare, which already cover recommended vaccines. The burden of the mandate would fall most heavily on insurers that do not currently provide vaccine benefits because they would have to develop new programs to do so.

Legislative action would be required to implement the proposed mandate and to authorize reimbursement payments. Such legislation should include both ERISA and ERISA-exempt plans to achieve a universal standard of vaccine coverage in all private health plans. Additional regulatory action would be required to ensure that the mandate applied to those vaccines designated as high priority primarily on the basis of their spillover effects.

The Subsidy Plan. The committee recommends that the government replace existing vaccine purchase programs with an insurance mandate funded by a new federal finance plan that includes a subsidy, reimbursement, and voucher arrangement. The subsidy amount for each vaccine in the program would be derived from a calculation of the societal benefit of the vaccine. The funded mandate would have the following features:

- All health insurers (both public and private) would purchase recommended vaccines for children and adults or delegate that responsibility to their participating providers.
- Insurers would be required to furnish recommended vaccines to their providers or reimburse their providers at least the purchase price they paid, up to the federal subsidy amount.

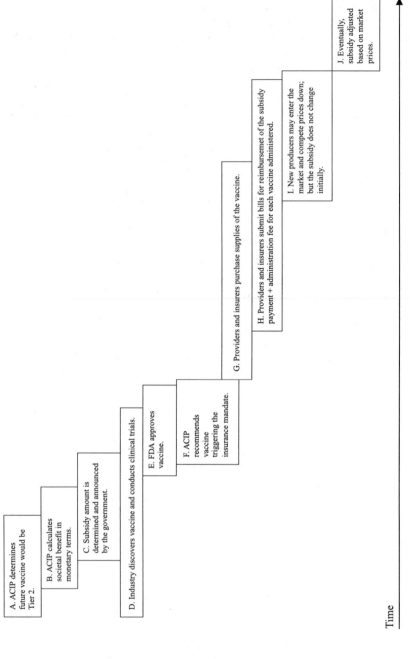

A. ACIP determines future vaccine would be Tier 2.

B. ACIP calculates societal benefit in monetary terms.

C. Subsidy amount is determined and announced by the government.

D. Industry discovers vaccine and conducts clinical trials.

E. FDA approves vaccine.

F. ACIP recommends vaccine triggering the insurance mandate.

G. Providers and insurers purchase supplies of the vaccine.

H. Providers and insurers submit bills for reimbursemet of the subsidy payment + administration fee for each vaccine administered.

I. New producers may enter the market and compete prices down; but the subsidy does not change initially.

J. Eventually, subsidy adjusted based on market prices.

Time

FIGURE 7-1 Proposed new vaccine development and subsidy process.

NOTES:

A. ACIP first identifies those diseases for which vaccines would be feasible and desirable. This hypothetical example uses respiratory syncytial virus (RSV) to illustrate the mechanics of the committee's proposed financing approach. In this example, an effective RSV vaccine is determined to qualify as a Tier 2 candidate for development because of its highly communicable nature and its toll in terms of morbidity, mortality, and economic costs. According to a recent study, RSV is associated with an average of more than 17,000 deaths per year, mainly among the elderly and young children (Thompson et al., 2003).

B and C. ACIP calculates societal benefit as described in detail in Figure 7-1. Based on that calculation, the government sets and announces a subsidy amount, in advance, to stimulate development of the vaccine by industry.

D and E. Steps B and C shorten the time required for discovery, development, licensure, and release of an RSV vaccine.

F. Improved coordination between FDA and ACIP results in quick approval of the new vaccine for use among infants and the elderly. This also triggers the coverage mandate.

G and H. Supplies of the vaccine are purchased by providers, insurers, and others, and government reimbursement for the vaccines that are administered begins.

I and J. Other producers may enter the market when the patent expires or production licenses are granted. The subsidy, in fact, encourages other companies to develop competing products. While this may reduce prices paid by physicians and insurers, the subsidy amount will remain high for some additional period, resulting in a windfall profit for physicians, insurers, or other vaccine purchasers. Eventually, the subsidy will be allowed to move toward the market price.

- Insurers would bill the federal government for the vaccines purchased or reimbursed. The government would reimburse all public and private health plans for vaccine purchases and administration fees through a central billing office located within the U.S. Department of Health and Human Services. The payment office would ensure that federal reimbursement fees were consistent with the level of subsidy and that the vaccines fell within the coverage mandates established by ACIP under recommendation 2 below.

The Value of the Subsidy. Using a subsidy rather than an administered price has certain key advantages. The subsidy would shift discussion away from the costs of production (which are not known) and price, and focus attention on the societal benefits of selected vaccine products. Thus, when policy makers determined health budgets for vaccines, they could compare the benefits of one product against those of another in terms of the public health goals they wished to achieve. The subsidy approach would also encourage policy makers to ask whether existing resources are adequate to achieve immunization goals. Second, the subsidy approach would make more transparent the implicit assumptions that already guide vaccine recommendations and purchasing negotiations. Third, a subsidy strategy could cause the vaccine industry to become more productive by creating incentives to invest in vaccines that have higher societal benefits than others. Finally, the subsidy approach would offer companies greater certitude that their investments in the development and production of vaccines having significant societal benefits will be adequately compensated.

If instead of a subsidy approach the government purchased all vaccines for a negotiated price, there would be no market basis for determining an appropriate price in the long run, and prices could become subject to political influence. The subsidy approach preserves some aspects of the market. It uses a formula method for setting the subsidy that is constant across all vaccines and is less subject to political manipulation. As a result, it reduces the uncertainty regarding future government-set prices that constrains industry investment in R&D.

The prospect of a guaranteed market for selected vaccines would produce incentives for manufacturers to invest in the clinical trial, licensing, and production processes that are necessary to move a vaccine product from the early stage of discovery to its use in routine medical care. In the past, private investments in vaccine production have been influenced not only by the regulatory costs of bringing a new product to market but also by uncertainties about the size of the public market and the discounts to be negotiated by the government.

Therefore, the Secretary of Health and Human Services should establish a fixed dollar subsidy that the government is willing to support based on an assessment of each vaccine's efficacy and value, and guarantee that the government will be willing to pay that subsidy as soon as one or more vaccines are available for use. The committee offers the following guidelines for determining the formula to be used in setting the subsidy amount:

- ACIP (or some other independent advisory body) should conduct an analysis to determine the monetary value to society of each vaccine. Definitions and estimates of societal benefit should be comprehensive and include a broad range of costs that extend beyond direct health care savings, such as longevity, quality of life, and reductions in caregiver burden. Societal benefit, as defined by this committee, is a measure of the total benefits provided by a vaccine, including both private benefits accruing to individuals who are immunized and benefits to others from a reduced likelihood of contracting a disease. Box 7-1 describes a generic process for calculating the societal benefit of a vaccine.
- Vaccines traditionally have been recognized as having substantial spillover effects since immunization protects not just the individual, but also others in society, from contagious diseases. This is not equally true of all vaccines, however. For example, tetanus vaccine, while highly beneficial, is mainly a private good. Tetanus is not easily transmitted and therefore does not substantially affect the health of others. Some new vaccines currently in development, such as therapeutic cancer vaccines, share this characteristic. The subsidy should apply principally only to vaccines that have strong spillover effects, that is, vaccines that protect against highly contagious infectious diseases and meet other criteria established by ACIP (see recommendation 2 below).
- The federal subsidy should be some percentage (no more than 100 percent) of the monetary value of the societal benefit of the vaccines that meet these criteria. This percentage should be based on a formula that is applied consistently across all such vaccines for some fixed period of years. A subsidy of less than 100 percent of societal benefit is justified in that some of that benefit accrues to the individual receiving a vaccine. On the other hand, low subsidies coupled with a mandate for vaccine benefits could lead to higher numbers of uninsured persons.
- The fixed-price subsidy would function as an incentive for successful development of future vaccines. An incentive, though smaller, may also be desirable to maintain producer interest in currently licensed vaccines and to encourage improvements in their manufacture, efficacy, safety, storage, and administration. The subsidy for currently licensed vaccines would be set in a different manner. The committee is not prepared to recommend a specific formula but advises that the subsidy be based on recent private-sector prices, be no higher than the calculated societal

---

BOX 7-1
Calculating the Societal Benefits of Vaccines

The calculation of societal benefits for a vaccine in advance is based on a highly developed cost–benefit/effectiveness/utility research literature (IOM, 2000b; Miller and Hinman, 1999). While technical issues must be addressed, the feasibility of the cost–benefit approach has been established through a wide range of economic studies involving vaccines and other medical interventions (Jacobs and Meyerhoff, 2001; McGuire, 2003). The committee's notion of societal benefit includes three type of benefits:

- Medical costs that are averted by reducing the incidence of disease
- Nonmonetary benefits, such as years of life and quality of life
- Indirect benefits, such as increased productivity

Calculating medical costs requires estimates of the disease incidence without the vaccine and the health care expenditures that would result from treatment of the disease, such as hospitalizations, physician visits, home health visits, nursing home stays, and drugs. For diseases currently without a vaccine, substantial data exist on treatment costs and disease incidence.

The calculation of nonmonetary benefits can draw on a substantial literature that suggests monetary values for years of life gained. Quality-of-life and disability measurements are also standard in the literature. Using a common standard across each analysis is critical so that comparisons can be made across different vaccines. Finally, indirect benefits include such factors as increased productivity and reduced burden on family caregivers.

Certain costs, such as adverse reactions to vaccines or the additional time costs associated with vaccination, should be subtracted from the total benefits of vaccines. Also, the stream of future benefits and costs must be discounted to the present. The final net benefit amount divided by the number of people to be vaccinated is the calculated societal benefit on which the subsidy would be based.

Issues and controversies abound in the calculation of these values. A number of these issues are summarized in the report of the Panel on Cost-Effectiveness in Medicine and Health (Gold et al., 1996). Assumptions required by the calculation—e.g., variables to include; valuations of life, disability, and morbidity; and the discount rate—must be made by a consensus panel or regulatory body with a substantial degree of expert input.

benefit, and include an annual adjustment based on inflation and significant production cost factors (such as changes in regulatory requirements).

• Under the proposed approach, the federal subsidy includes a clinician fee for the administration of vaccines. The committee suggests that the Centers for Medicare and Medicaid Services (CMS) determine differential clinician fees for childhood and adult vaccines, as well as for other significant cost-related categories, through the Resource-Based Relative Value Scale (RBRVS) process, and that these rates be included in the total amount of the subsidy.

The Voucher Plan. Under the proposed strategy, uninsured children and high-risk adults would be enrolled within a national vaccination voucher program. The committee considered two options for the voucher payment. Under one option, each child and adult would be provided with an electronic card certifying, for each specified vaccine, the amount the clinician will be reimbursed for the vaccine cost and administration fee. The voucher card would be presented to the clinician, who would bill the government for those amounts. The creation of a central or community-based registry for vouchers and immunization records would allow clinicians to update records and assist in the replacement of lost cards. This option would create an administrative expense for the government but would relieve the physician of the burden of verifying eligibility at the point of service. This approach would also reduce missed opportunities and referrals and encourage greater participation by physicians in the national immunization system. The eligibility determination component could be tied to existing programs, such as Medicaid, to reduce the administrative burden.

A second option is to allow each clinician to bill the government for reimbursement of uninsured persons without requiring individual documentation. The central billing office would determine eligibility and draw the reimbursement from the appropriate fund (e.g., if the patient were insured, the payment to that insurer would be debited). This approach would be feasible under a universal coverage approach, since the government would ultimately pay every claim. It would be more problematic for the adult component of the committee's proposal, which applies only to the high-risk subset of the adult population.

Advantages. The committee's proposed strategy has several clear advantages. It would:

• Improve incentives for the development of new vaccines by providing manufacturers with assurance of adequate pricing and returns for those vaccines that confer substantial public benefit.

- Increase immunization rates by eliminating or reducing barriers to access associated with vaccine costs or health insurance benefits.
- Create a more pluralistic market for vaccines that would encourage providers and health plans to purchase vaccines best suited to the needs of their patients and subscribers.
- Build upon the strengths of the current arrangements of public and private health plans and avoid the creation of separate or parallel programs. The proposed finance plan offers an opportunity to improve national immunization rates over those achieved during the past decade. By reducing the likelihood of missed opportunities based on eligibility requirements or insurance plan benefits, the plan would enable more individuals to receive vaccines as part of routine health care services. The barrier of high deductibles or copayments for recommended vaccines would be eliminated for disadvantaged children and adults.
- Eliminate the economic distortions and administrative barriers associated with the direct federal purchase of vaccines. The government currently purchases 52–55 percent of all childhood vaccines and has substantial monopsony power over vaccine prices. The committee believes the continued availability of current and future vaccines is more likely to be assured if such market power is reduced. The committee's proposal would eliminate government price constraints and allow prices to move to levels that would be neither too low to stimulate investment by manufacturers nor so high as to constrain demand or limit availability.
- Reduce the role of government in purchasing vaccines and avoid delays now associated with eligibility standards, protracted contract negotiations, price caps, discretionary funding cycles, and discount arrangements. Gaps, delays, and disruptions in the vaccine delivery system occur as a result of the fragmented finance system and government contract negotiations for bulk purchases. Financing of vaccine purchases is disrupted by many factors: the lack of predictability of new vaccine approvals, delays in the negotiation of CDC vaccine contracts, problems associated with predicting the uptake rates of vaccines, and the time required to appropriate new discretionary funds through the state and federal budget processes. As a result, funding—even for vaccines that are part of the federal entitlement—may not be available when needed. The combination of the elimination of federal purchasing and access to federal funding for every vaccine covered by the subsidy would minimize the fragmentation problem.
- Reduce the potential for insurers and providers to shift the increasing costs of vaccines to individuals through high deductibles or copayments.
- Support the administration of vaccines within individuals' medical homes and strengthen the bond between immunization and other pri-

mary health care services. The finance plan should encourage the participation of both public and private health care providers in choosing vaccines that best meet the needs of the populations they serve. It should also reduce the administrative burden associated with ordering and maintaining different stockpiles of vaccine products on the basis of vaccine eligibility requirements.

• Support the rapid uptake of new recommended vaccines and reduce the disparities and fragmentation now associated with time delays involved in negotiating contracts and budgets for federal vaccine purchases. The finance plan would offer manufacturers strong incentives for interruption-free production and vaccine development while also controlling the costs of vaccine products. Once a vaccine had been approved, suppliers would be free to market their products directly to providers or health plans in a manner similar to that for pharmaceutical products. It is also presumed that higher vaccine prices would encourage additional investments in new vaccines providing societal benefit.

• Sustain the partnership among governments (federal, state, and local), health plans and health care providers, and vaccine companies in achieving the societal benefits of disease prevention. The current vaccine purchasing system (VFC and the Section 317 program) has stimulated thousands of community partnerships and public health linkages (e.g., state–provider collaborations in delivery, monitoring, and assessment systems). The proposed strategy seeks to sustain these partnerships by enhancing opportunities for public and private health plans to exchange information about immunization levels, community outreach efforts, assessments of clinician records, and other activities as part of their reimbursement requests. The central purpose of the strategy is to support a strong national immunization system and public access to vaccines while reducing the role of government in directly purchasing and distributing vaccine products. It is essential that the partnerships associated with earlier vaccine purchase arrangements be maintained and strengthened during the transition period while the new vaccine payment plan is being implemented.

• Maintain a market-oriented pricing approach. A key difference between the subsidy approach and a universal purchase approach is in the way prices are determined. The subsidy preserves important market features. Furthermore, it provides a formula-based method for price setting that is less subject to political manipulation and would be more acceptable to manufacturers.

Disadvantages. The committee recognizes that certain disadvantages are associated with the proposed vaccine payment system. The replacement of a government purchase price with a federal subsidy could result in higher prices for some vaccine products. The addition of new vaccines would also increase federal expenditures, although the degree of escalation under a subsidy arrangement (in lieu of government price negotiations) is not certain. These expenditures need to be balanced against future cost offsets that could occur as a result of savings due to the prevention of disease, as well as the benefits associated with future investments and innovation in vaccine production and development. Increases in expenditures would be limited by two considerations: (1) the insurance mandate and subsidy would apply only to certain vaccines—those that have significant spillover effects because they prevent highly contagious diseases, and (2) the societal value calculation represents a ceiling above which the insurance mandate, subsidy, and voucher would not apply.

The federal government currently spends about $1 billion annually to purchase vaccines through the VFC program and an additional $300 million (estimated) to purchase vaccines on behalf of state governments for distribution through the Section 317 program. These funds are allocated for the direct purchase of vaccines at discount prices. The proposed payment system would shift the entire burden of vaccine payments for children and high-risk adults (estimated to be about $2–3 billion in 2002) to the federal government while reducing the amount paid privately by health plans. This public expenditure could be expected to grow with the addition of new and more expensive vaccines to the recommended immunization schedule. Although some cost offsets could be expected (such as the personnel costs associated with the administration of current vaccine purchase programs in state and federal agencies), these offsets would not be large.

In addition, federal vaccine expenditures, even in a universal program, would remain substantially lower than other medical costs already subsidized by the federal government. Furthermore, because the price would never exceed the subsidy amount, which would be at or below the value of the vaccine to society, the vaccine would always be worth funding up to that price.[2]

There are many competing uses for public funds, both within health care budgets and between health care budgets and other governmental programs. While the increased burden of the proposed plan on the public sector appears to be justifiable in the interests of both public health and

---

[2]At least one vaccine, pneumococcal conjugate, may already be priced above the dollar value of its societal benefit (Jacobs and Meyerhoff, 2001). This vaccine would be grandfathered under a separate calculation used for all currently recommended vaccines as described in recommendation 1.

investment in the production of vaccines that meet criteria for societal benefit, the significant budgetary increases for vaccine payments need to be acknowledged and planned for in projecting health care costs.

Second, setting a subsidy for vaccines not yet licensed based on a calculation of societal benefit, without reference to market forces, involves significant challenges.[3,4] These include defining and assigning a measurable value for the societal benefits of vaccines and calculating the level of subsidy necessary to achieve the goals of assuring access to vaccines and rewarding innovation. The calculation of societal benefit would require the development of a consistent methodology to resolve numerous technical difficulties. Controversies could arise in assigning monetary values to life-years and quality of life as part of the societal benefit calculations.

Substantial expert guidance and public debate could be required to resolve these controversies.[5]

Potential pitfalls include the risk that policy makers would overestimate the level of subsidy necessary to stimulate production and innovation, thus offering higher-than-necessary prices for vaccines. Or the subsidy could underestimate the levels necessary to compensate manufacturers for their investments, thus discouraging the production and distribution of vaccines that have important societal benefits.

The committee believes the resolution of these concerns will require extensive discussion and deliberation with major stakeholders (see recommendation 3, below). At the most fundamental level, certain key questions remain, which are addressed later in this section: Given the uncertainties associated with calculating the value of certain types of societal benefits and uncertainties about the marginal cost of producing, distributing and delivering a vaccine, should the subsidy be bounded so that, for example, the price of a new vaccine could not exceed some multiple of existing vaccine prices? Should recommendations vary according to the

---

[3]This discussion draws on an analysis originally presented in an earlier report on education finance, prepared by the National Research Council (NRC) (Ladd and Hansen, 1999). In this study, the NRC committee recommends that the emerging concept of "adequacy" be used to finance educational programs in order to focus attention on sufficiency of funding for desired educational outcomes. Both that report and the present study highlight the importance of aligning finance systems with societal goals and benefits while recognizing the technical challenges involved in doing so.

[4]One committee member argued that setting a subsidy in advance on the basis of calculated societal benefit could be unnecessary and excessively difficult and could result in unnecessarily high prices.

[5]The technical difficulties associated with calculating societal benefits and with achieving political agreement on critical value assumptions, such as the monetary value of a life-year, are explored by the Panel on Cost-Effectiveness in Health and Medicine (Gold et al., 1996).

price of a vaccine? Should manufacturers be required to disclose development and production costs as part of the subsidy plan? How should the subsidy be applied to early versions of vaccines that may have unresolved safety concerns or side effects?

These are not technical questions for which scientific answers can be provided; they require difficult political judgments and social choices that need to be informed by public discussion. Thus at some level, assigning values to vaccine benefits necessarily becomes subjective. Government would have to make key assumptions—for example, about the monetary value of life—that could change over time in response to budgetary pressures or new political or regulatory regimes. Pharmaceutical companies would likely realize this and thus might not respond favorably to higher prices based on this scheme. However, such assumptions are already implicit in current ACIP and government purchasing policy for vaccines. The committee's recommended approach would require that these assumptions be made explicit, lending greater transparency to the decision-making process.

Finally, implementation of the committee's proposal would be legislatively complex. The creation of a new government payment and voucher plan would require substantial legislative action, including amendments to established law in a variety of areas (e.g., ERISA, Public Health Act, Medicare, Medicaid, SCHIP). The need for review and action across multiple congressional committee jurisdictions involves inherent risks of piecemeal adoption unless a comprehensive legislative plan can be developed that has strong bipartisan support. While particular stakeholder groups (the vaccine industry, health insurers, or physicians) might support or oppose certain components of the proposed strategy, a broad-based approach would need to be crafted that could achieve common goals, avoid special interests, and help define the basic incentives that should guide federal policy for vaccine finance. Table 7-1 summarizes the legislative impact of the committee's recommendations.

Recommendation 2: The Secretary of the Department of Health and Human Services should propose changes in the procedures and membership of ACIP so that its recommendations can associate vaccine coverage decisions with societal benefits and costs, including consideration of the impact of the price of a vaccine on recommendations for its use.

The Secretary of DHHS should develop rules that address both the ACIP membership and decision-making process. These rules would modify current practices through administrative action or legislation, where necessary.

TABLE 7-1 Legislative Impact of Committee Recommendations

Recommendation	Relevant Laws and Areas for Legislative Consideration
Make federal immunization coverage mandate applicable to all forms of public and private health insurance. Establish coverage levels in accordance with the ACIP recommendations.	• ERISA (29 U.S.C. §1001 et seq.): all ERISA-covered employee health benefit plans • Public Health Service Act (42 U.S.C. §300-gg et seq.): state-regulated insurance • Federal employee health benefits (5 U.S.C. §8901 et seq.) • U.S. postal workers (39 U.S.C. §1005) • Health insurance for members of the armed forces (10 U.S.C. §1071 et seq.) • Medicare (42 U.S.C. §1395 et seq.) • Medicaid (42 U.S.C. §1396 et seq.) • State Children's Health Insurance Plan (SCHIP) (42 U.S.C. §1397 et seq.) • Veterans Administration (38 U.S. C. §1701 et seq.)[a] • Indian Health Service (25 U.S.C. §1621 et seq.)[a]
Establish new federal subsidy for insurance plans to cover vaccine benefits. Establish new federal voucher program for all ACIP-recommended vaccines for all individuals who are uninsured.	• New legislation as needed
Restructure ACIP with respect to membership and decision-making process used to establish the recommended vaccine schedule, including adoption of "tiered" recommendations for mandated insurance benefits.	• New legislation as needed pursuant to the authority of the DHHS Secretary's general advisory committee (42 U.S. C. §217a)
Restructure the VFC program and National Vaccine Program as necessary to conform to new coverage mechanisms.	• Amendments as needed to VFC (42 U.S.C. §1396d(r)) and the National Vaccine Program (42 U.S.C. §247)

[a]Technically, neither program is insurance. However, both are major sources of third-party financing for basic medical care, and both furnish immunizations.

With regard to ACIP membership, voting membership should be expanded to include expertise in health insurance benefit design, public and private health care delivery systems, consumer issues (including concerns regarding vulnerable populations such as disabled persons, racial and ethnic minorities, and rural populations), health economics and finance, cost–

benefit assessment, and vaccine manufacturing. The representation of these perspectives is essential to inform ACIP decision making with respect to the impact of vaccine price and coverage on population groups, providers, payors, and other key stakeholders. At the same time, it is important to maintain the independence and balance that have traditionally guided ACIP recommendation procedures through a rigorous and transparent conflict and bias screening process for voting members. Current employees or agents of firms within the insurance and vaccine manufacturing industries should not participate as voting members, although access to their expertise is necessary to inform committee deliberations.

With respect to general vaccine recommendations, ACIP should continue its present practice of recommending current and new vaccines for universal or selected populations within the immunization schedule. These determinations should be based on a vaccine's efficacy, safety, cost-effectiveness (reflecting current price information), feasibility, supply, and other considerations.

With regard to mandate and subsidy determinations, ACIP should carry out an additional process to determine whether a vaccine has sufficient spillover effects to warrant its inclusion in the new insurance mandate and subsidy category. The mandate determination for new vaccines would require a judgment about the extent to which a vaccine offers societal benefits beyond its value to the vaccinated individual. An important criterion in determining societal benefits should be the extent to which immunization conveys herd immunity, whereby immunization of some individuals offers protection to others who have not been vaccinated or have insufficient immunity to prevent transmission. The mandate would apply principally to vaccines with substantial spillover effects. However, other vaccines, such as therapeutic vaccines, would be considered for inclusion in cases of exceptional societal benefit, particularly when disparities in immunization rates between insured and uninsured persons persisted for a substantial time after licensure of the vaccine.

Once a vaccine had been selected for inclusion under the insurance mandate as discussed in recommendation 1 above, ACIP would calculate the monetary value of the federal subsidy for reimbursement to public and private insurers. This calculation would be based on a methodology that would assign values to such factors as reduced health expenditures, enhanced quality of life, and increased labor productivity.

The mandate and subsidy process would apply to both current and future vaccines. Future vaccines should receive primary consideration to stimulate the development of new vaccine products. Current ACIP-recommended vaccine components, such as tetanus, could be "grandfathered" into the mandate and subsidy category to avoid confusion and disruptions to the current vaccine schedule and immunization system.

Staff support for these new functions and the redesigned ACIP would require expansion of the supporting responsibilities of the National Vaccine Policy Office and the National Immunization Program within CDC.

Table 7-2 illustrates the existing ACIP procedure and contrasts it with the new, enhanced procedure that is recommended by the committee. The existing procedure is represented by blocks A and B (current). ACIP decides whether to recommend each vaccine for universal use (block A) or use by a targeted subset of the population (block B). Its recommendations are based on a range of factors, including cost-effectiveness. ACIP also makes *permissive* recommendations, which means that providers should use their judgment in deciding whether to vaccinate based on individual patients' risk factors. A separate vote determines whether the vaccine will be included in the VFC entitlement program.

Under the committee's proposed procedure—blocks A and B (new)— ACIP would continue to make Tier 1 recommendations. But in addition to considering a vaccine's cost-effectiveness, ACIP would conduct (or commission) an analysis to calculate the monetary value of the societal benefit of the vaccine, providing a pricing benchmark to be included among the factors considered by ACIP in determining its recommendation. Also, ACIP would no longer vote on inclusion in the VFC entitlement program since the new system would replace that program.

If a vaccine received a Tier 1 recommendation, ACIP would make a separate Tier 2 determination as to whether the vaccine should be included in the mandate and subsidy categories (blocks C and D). A new vaccine might be recommended for addition to the schedule (Tier 1) but not be included in the government mandate and subsidy program because it lacked significant spillover effects so that its benefits accrue primarily to the individual rather than to society as a whole (an example would be a vaccine that prevents diabetes or cancer). Individual health care providers could still purchase and administer the vaccine, and health plans could voluntarily include it as a benefit. But health plans would not be required to include the vaccine in their benefits package, and a government subsidy would not be available to reimburse the cost of the vaccine to health care providers. A vaccine might also receive a restricted recommendation to the mandate and subsidy program, for example, limiting a high-priced or less cost-effective vaccine to selected high-risk populations (block D).

Under the committee's proposed approach, ACIP would also consider future vaccines that were not yet available but could be beneficial to the public's health. Such vaccines would bypass the usual schedule recommendation process (until they had actually been developed and licensed) and go directly to the Tier 2 mandate recommendation process. Vaccines

TABLE 7-2 Proposed Redesign of ACIP Recommendations

Tier	Feature	Notes	Universal Population	Targeted Population
Tier 1	Current Procedure	• Consideration of efficacy, safety, feasibility, supply, cost-effectiveness • Full and permissive recommendations • VFC vote	A (current)	B (current)
	New Procedure	• Consideration of efficacy, safety, feasibility, supply, cost-effectiveness • Full and permissive recommendations • Calculation of societal benefit • Formal consideration of price data, if available • Elimination of VFC vote	A (new)	B (new)
Tier 2	Mandate	• Selection of vaccines with substantial public benefits and spillover effects • Current recommended vaccines grandfathered • Selective consideration of vaccines with limited spillover effects	C	D
	Subsidy Calculation	• Based on the value of calculated societal benefit • Consistently applied formula • Incentive for development of not-yet-licensed vaccines • Different formula for current vaccines, based on former prices with adjustments for significant cost factors	E	F

currently recommended would be included automatically—i.e., grand-fathered—in the mandate and subsidy program.

Once an existing or future vaccine had been recommended for the mandate and subsidy program, ACIP would determine and publish a sub-sidy amount (blocks E and F) that the government would agree to pro-vide as described in recommendation 1.

Recommendation 3: As part of the implementation of recommendations 1 and 2, the National Vaccine Program Office should convene a series of stakeholder deliberations on the administrative, technical, and legislative issues associated with a shift from vaccine purchase to a vaccine mandate, subsidy, and voucher finance strategy. In addition, the Centers for Disease Control and Prevention (CDC) should sponsor a postimplementation evaluation study (in 5 years, for example). CDC should also initiate a research program aimed at improving the measurement of the societal value of vaccines, addressing methodological challenges, and providing a basis for comparing the impact of different measurement approaches in achieving national immunization goals.

Recommendations 1 and 2 represent a significant departure from current law and practice. A change of this magnitude is warranted to address the fundamental and systemic problems that confront the national immunization system. Piecemeal changes are unlikely to solve these problems. Incremental reforms also are incapable of achieving an appropriate balance between access and availability in vaccine financing.

In formulating its recommendations, the committee has sketched the broad outlines of long-term strategic reforms. These recommendations do not address all aspects of the shift from the existing vaccine purchase programs to a mandate, subsidy, and voucher plan; nor do they incorporate the comprehensive legislative agenda that would be necessary to achieve these reforms. A major national debate and examination of the committee's proposals among diverse stakeholders is necessary prior to full implementation of these recommendations,

The magnitude and complexity of the mandate, voucher, and subsidy recommendations presented above are significant, and the recommendations would be difficult to implement. A financing strategy designed both to achieve higher levels of access to vaccines and to encourage the process of innovation would introduce a greater level of administrative complexity into the national immunization system. The National Vaccine Program Office, in collaboration with CDC, should foster a sustained dialogue regarding the best methods for estimating the societal value of new vaccines and for achieving a balance between access and innovation through vaccine financing strategies.

The committee recommends that the National Vaccine Program Office convene a series of regional and national meetings on vaccine finance as part of the implementation process. These meetings should highlight areas of administrative uncertainty (such as the treatment of therapeutic vaccines or the handling of copayments under an insurance mandate for vaccines) and methodological challenges (such as the treatment of labor market activity in the assessment of social value), as well as identify strategies that can inform the implementation of the recommended vaccine mandate, subsidy, and voucher system. The meetings should include representation from all sectors affected by the proposed shifts in policies and practices: public health agencies, health insurers (both public and private), health care providers, employers, industry, and consumers.

Implementation Plan. The deliberations convened by the National Vaccine Program Office could examine more fully the administrative complexity of individual components of the committee's recommendations and explore strategies that could help reduce areas of uncertainty or potential unintended consequences. These deliberations should address how the proposed arrangements might be implemented through a staged rollout that would be informed by further data and analysis. Topics to be addressed within these discussions include the following:

What populations should be included in the vaccine payment plan? The federal vaccine payment plan is envisioned primarily as a means of addressing the immunization needs of young children, older adults, and high-risk adults between the ages of 18 and 65. The inclusion of other populations—such as all adolescents (under age 21) and all adults, regardless of their health condition—should be considered as well. The initial purpose of the expanded coverage is to target public finance toward those who are currently underserved. A second goal, which supports the proposal for universal coverage of all children and adults, is to reduce the current fragmentation in vaccine coverage that leads to gaps and administrative burdens in determining eligibility and to foster efficiency in providing access to vaccines that are delivered primarily in private health care settings. The means by which vaccines would be delivered to and reimbursed for different groups might differ by age, employment circumstances, and access to health care services.

How would the insurance mandate and subsidy system operate? The insurance mandate would apply to all public and private insurers, including Medicaid, SCHIP, Medicare, and other public insurance (such as CHAMPUS) and public health programs (such as that of the Indian Health Service), as well as both state-regulated insurance plans and self-funded employer plans (which are exempt from state regulation under the Employee Retirement Income Security Act [ERISA]). The mandate would extend to all insured persons within these health plans. The voucher system would provide access to vaccines for all uninsured people in these categories. For most public programs, current program funding for vaccine purchases and vaccine administration would be replaced by the vaccine payment system dollars. For example, vaccines administered through Medicaid and SCHIP would no longer be funded through those programs' federal–state matching funds but through the new centralized vaccine system. In contrast, Medicare would be included in the mandate but would pay for immunizations through its own program funds for purposes of administrative efficiency.

How should societal value be calculated? The committee defines the societal value of a vaccine as its total benefits, including both the private benefits to the person receiving it and the benefits to others. Using this approach, a monetary value is assigned to all benefits associated with a new vaccine that can be determined and measured (for example, future medical costs that are averted, as well as additional life-years and enhanced quality of life). The sum of these values represents the vaccine's societal benefit. As noted above in the discussion of disadvantages, this calculation involves certain technical challenges. Developing a consistent methodology and making assumptions explicit for all vaccines would be of value in the decision-making process not only for vaccines but in other spheres of health care as well.

The committee recognizes that the subsidy amount for vaccines would be sensitive to key assumptions about what should be included in societal benefit calculations. Cost-effectiveness analyses (CEAs) and cost–benefit analyses (CBAs) have been conducted on vaccines and in other areas of medicine for decades, utilizing a range of methodologies. The costs and benefits included in these studies, and the methodologies for measuring them and incorporating them into the analyses, vary widely from study to study and involve some fundamental disagreements about what should and should not be included.

In 1993, a nonfederal panel of experts in CEA and CBA—the Panel on Cost-Effectiveness in Health and Medicine—was convened by the U.S. Public Health Service to consider issues related to the definition and measurement of costs, benefits, and levels of effectiveness in CEA and CBA studies. The panel's report, which was released in 1996 (Gold et al., 1996), enumerates a wide range of issues on which disagreements exist regarding the design of these studies. The list of issues on which further consensus needs to be achieved includes the following: Should costs include only health care costs for the drug and "related" medical services? Should costs include all changes in subsequent medical costs, including the additional health care costs of patients who will now live longer? Should they include future consumption of any good or service? If so, should future productivity or work effort be netted out of that amount? Which time and labor costs to patients and employers should be included—time spent seeking care, absenteeism, withdrawal from the labor force due to the employee's own health or the need to address problems of family members? Should loss of productivity of coworkers due to team efforts, friction costs associated with temporary substitution of workers with less firm- and task-specific skills, and shifts in on-the-job productivity be included? If such time or labor market effects are included, which wage rates should be used? Should market wages be adjusted for gender, racial, and ethnic disparities? How should time costs be valued for children, the disabled, or the retired, who have no wage to use as a benchmark? This is only a partial list of the issues raised by the panel.

The mandate and subsidy approach recommended by the committee requires that benefits and costs be calculated to determine the total societal benefit, which becomes the basis for a monetary subsidy. To establish vaccine subsidy amounts in a consistent manner, it is essential that a standard methodology for measuring costs and benefits be established and followed. Currently, every CEA or CBA study incorporates assumptions, either implicitly or explicitly, regarding each of these issues. While consistency within the literature may be increasing, there is still substantial variation in the assumptions applied. The Panel on Cost-Effectiveness in Health and Medicine established the notion that each analysis should formulate a "reference case" using a common set of assumptions on some of these key issues, but the panel stopped short of recommending what the standard assumptions should be. To establish a consistent approach to the determination of societal benefit across the range of current and future vaccines, these assumptions will have to be made and be applied consistently.

The committee envisions that ACIP or some other independent body, or an office within CDC, would make these determinations, with expert guidance from leading researchers in the field of CEA and CBA. Some of these decisions may be controversial, such as the methodologies used to assign monetary value to life-years or improvements in quality of life, especially among different age or disability groups, and differences between the social and individual valuations of preventive versus critical care. Decisions regarding the methodologies that should be employed are too technical for this committee to have addressed them in this report. But the committee does suggest that in resolving these issues, the determining body strongly weight current accepted practice among leading, mainstream practitioners in the field of medical CEA and CBA, rather than rely on novel approaches and measurement methodologies. In addition, recognizing that the field is evolving, this body should consider changes in assumptions, the inclusion of additional economic variables, and changes in measurement methodologies over time. As changes in the standard methodology were adopted, however, they would have to be incorporated retroactively into all studies to maintain consistency across all vaccines.

How would the calculated societal benefit be used to determine the subsidy amount? For not-yet-licensed vaccines, the creation of a predetermined subsidy is intended to be an incentive to stimulate private-sector investment in vaccine development. Determining the amount of the subsidy would require a calculation of the societal benefit of each future vaccine, but the value of the subsidy would not necessarily equal the full value of the societal benefit. While the subsidy should not exceed the societal value of the vaccine product, it should also not be so low that it fails to serve as an adequate incentive for research and development. Different approaches might be considered, such as adopting a fixed standard (for example, 90 percent of the societal value) or limiting the range of new vaccine prices to some multiple of current prices.

How would the subsidy for current vaccines be determined? For current or newly licensed vaccines, the subsidy calculation would require consideration of both the societal value of the vaccine product and recent market prices. Some vaccines might receive a subsidy significantly higher than current prices if judged to be undervalued in terms of their societal benefit. Adjustments in the value of the subsidy might also be warranted to account for inflation, as well as changes in the costs of production or regulatory compliance.

Who would administer the subsidy and voucher system? The vaccine payment system is designed to serve multiple objectives: to address the vaccine needs of vulnerable populations, to assure a reliable supply of current and future vaccines by diversifying the vaccine purchasing market, and to relieve clinicians of the administrative burden of determining individual eligibility for vaccines. Ideally, one federal agency within DHHS would be responsible for administering both the subsidy and the voucher system, as well as regulating compliance with the insurance mandate for vaccine coverage. Certain responsibilities might be delegated to state agencies (in such areas as insurance regulation and administration of the voucher plan), but a central coordinating strategy would be required to assure consistent eligibility criteria and practices throughout the states.

How would the proposed mandate treat deductibles and copayments? While many states have mandated first-dollar coverage for vaccines, immunization costs might apply toward the general deductible that is customary practice for health plans. While many current vaccines are inexpensive, significant price increases can be expected in the future. Cost sharing could encourage consumers to shop for efficient providers and help control inflationary pressures; however, it could adversely affect immunization rates should financial factors become burdensome for the consumer. The extent to which cost sharing should be included in the vaccine payment plan would require further consideration in the implementation process.

Evaluation Plan. The positive and negative effects of replacing current safety net programs with the proposed government-funded mandate cannot be predicted with any degree of certainty. The VFC entitlement and Section 317 vaccine purchase program have been productive tools in improving immunization levels within the public sector. These programs have a history of strong bipartisan support and effective delivery of vaccines for disadvantaged populations, especially during difficult fiscal times, but are associated with disruptions in supply and a decrease in the number of vaccine manufacturers. Similarly, state-supported vaccine purchase programs are often the foundation for safety net immunization efforts in certain jurisdictions. Strategies need to be developed to assure that the payment system advocated here will at least sustain, and ideally improve, current immunization rates among disadvantaged populations. Given the uncertainties associated with the introduction of a new vaccine payment system, an evaluation study should be designed as part of the system's implementation.

In addition, the committee recommends that CDC organize an evaluation study 5 years following implementation to inform the new vaccine mandate, subsidy, and voucher system. Evaluation criteria should include the system's effects on government expenditures, access to vaccines within disadvantaged populations, and innovation within the vaccine industry. Its findings would form the basis for midcourse corrections in program design. Specifically, this study should include an analysis of the impact of the mandate and subsidy in two distinct areas: access to vaccines and the availability of the vaccine supply.

In the first area, data should be gathered on how the payment system affects the delivery of vaccines to selected population groups (insured, uninsured, and underinsured), age cohorts (young children and high-risk adults), and geographic settings (rural and urban), possibly through demonstration studies aimed at identifying key challenges involved in the implementation process in selected states. The costs of implementation, outreach, education, reimbursement, and oversight should be measured to determine how to gain greater efficiencies in administering the program.

In the second area, the impact of the diversified market and predetermined subsidy plan should be examined in light of their relationship to private investments in the production and licensing of new vaccine products. The evaluation study should consider the assumptions that guide the calculations of societal benefit, as well as other data that influence the level of vaccine subsidy and voucher payments.

Demonstration projects are often used to test a new approach prior to full implementation. In this case, however, it would be difficult or impossible to conduct a demonstration that could address a change in the structure of the national vaccine market, which is a central feature of the committee's proposal. Major programs are often implemented without empirical evidence indicating that they will succeed (as was indeed the case with VFC, Medicare, and Medicaid); rather, to the extent that such evidence is available, it typically only supports the need for the program.

Research Agenda. CDC should develop an ongoing research program to examine interactions among vaccine finance strategies, immunization rates in the public and private health sectors, and the pace of innovation in the vaccine industry. Addressing many of the issues raised in this report will require further understanding of the ways in which basic market forces interact with access to and the delivery of vaccines to children, adolescents, and adults. Limited data are available to support rigorous examination of such empirical questions as the relationship of insurance benefits to immunization status. More funding is needed to support research studies that can monitor the extent to which pricing, supply, mandates, and other health policy and health finance factors influence the performance and outcomes of immunization efforts. Suggested topics for an initial set of research studies include the following:

- The numbers and characteristics of children and adults having public or private insurance benefits that include immunization and the types of restrictions on their immunization benefits.
- The impact of insurance status (both public and private) and cost-sharing arrangements on the timing and setting of vaccine administration and immunization status.
- The impact of alternative vaccine payment arrangements on clinician behavior and referral rates for immunization.
- The effect of full or partial subsidies on the supply and delivery of childhood and adult vaccines.
- The relationship between vaccine prices and supplier investments in research and development.
- The relationship between U.S. and global vaccine production, supply, regulation, and prices.

FINAL OBSERVATIONS

The findings, alternative strategies, and recommendations set forth in this report provide a strategic blueprint to guide the nation's public and private health sectors in adapting to foreseeable changes in vaccine development in the decades ahead. The public and private partnership that supports the immunization of children and adults in the United States requires vigilance and flexibility in assuring that the social benefits of vaccines will continue to be available to all, regardless of ability to pay or health care setting. Assuring access and sustaining incentives that contribute to the availability of safe and effective vaccines are the twin goals that must guide vaccine finance strategies in the 21st century.

References

Abbotts, B., and L. Osborn. 1993. Immunization Status and Reasons for Immunization Delay Among Children Using Public Health Immunization Clinics. *American Journal of Diseases of Children* 147(9):965-968.

Academy for Health Services Research and Health Policy [AHSRHP]. 2001. *Understanding the Dynamics of "Crowd-Out": Defining Public/Private Coverage Substitution for Policy and Research.* Washington, DC: Academy for Health Services Research and Health Policy.

American Academy of Family Physicians. 2001. *Letter to the Centers for Medicare and Medicaid Services* (December 19).

American Academy of Pediatrics. 2001a. *Letter to the Centers for Medicare and Medicaid Services* (December 21).

_____. 2001b. *Letter to the Occupational Health and Safety Administration [OSHA]* (July 25).

_____. 2002. *Medicaid Reimbursement Survey, 2001: 50 States and the District of Columbia.* No date. Accessed online November 29, 2002 at http://www.aap.org/research/medreim PDF01/all_states.PDF.

_____. 2003. *Mandated Insurance Coverage of Childhood Vaccines* (March 8).

American Association of Health Plans. 2002. *Vaccine Purchasing Survey* (August).

American College of Physicians-American Society of Internal Medicine. 2001. *Letter to the Centers for Medicare and Medicaid Services* (September 26).

Arnould, R., and L. DeBrock. 1993. Equilibrium Outcomes in Vaccine Markets and the Implications for Policy Initiatives. In: *Supplying Vaccines: An Economic Analysis of Critical Issues.* Pauly, M., C. Robinson, S. Sepe, M. Sing, and M. Willian (eds.). London: IOS Press.

_____. 2002. *An Overview of the Market for Vaccines in the United States.* Unpublished. (Available from IOM.)

Aventis Pasteur. 2002. Aventis Pasteur. *Email Communication from C. Grant.* November 22. (Available from IOM.)

Bates, A., and F. Wolinsky. 1998. Personal, Financial, and Structural Barriers to Immunization in Socioeconomically Disadvantaged Urban Children. *Pediatrics* 101(4):591-596.

Batson, A. 2001. *Understanding the Vaccine Market and Its Economics: Obstacles and Potential Solutions.* Presentation to the Out of the Box Group, July 26, 2001.

Boyd, T., R. Linkins, K. Mason, I. Bulim, and B. Lemke. 2002. Assessing Immunization Registry Data Completeness in Bexar County, Texas. *American Journal of Preventive Medicine*
22(3):184-187.

Brichacek, A. 2001. Vaccine Worries. *Pharmaceutical Executive* 21.

Briss, P., S. Zaza, and M. Pappaioanou. 2000. Reviews of Evidence regarding Interventions
to Improve Vaccination Coverage in Children, Adolescents and Adults. *American Journal of Preventive Medicine* 18(1S):97-140.

Bureau of Labor Statistics. 2003. Tables from the *Current Population Survey, March 2001*. Email
from P. Willis, July 15. (Available from IOM.)

Butler, P. 2000. *ERISA and State Health Care Access Initiatives: Opportunities and Barriers*. New
York: The Commonwealth Fund.

Centers for Disease Control and Prevention. 1984. Diphtheria-Tetanus-Pertussis Vaccine
Shortage—United States. *Morbidity and Mortality Weekly Report* 33(49):695-696.

_____. 1991. Food and Drug Administration Approval of Use of Diphtheria and Tetanus
Toxoids and Acellular Pertussis Vaccine. *Morbidity and Mortality Weekly Report*
40(50):881-882.

_____. 1992. Acellular Pertussis Vaccine for Reinforcing and Booster Use B Supplementary
ACIP Statement. *Morbidity and Mortality Weekly Report* 41(RR-1):1-10.

_____. 1997. *United States Vaccine Research: A Delicate Fabric of Public and Private Collaboration*.
Accessed June 1, 2003. Available at: www.cdc.gov/od/nvpo/delfab.pdf.

_____. 1998. National, State, and Urban Area Vaccination Coverage Levels Among Children
Aged 19-35 Months—United States, July 1996-June 1997. *Morbidity and Mortality Weekly
Report* 47(6):108-116.

_____. 1999a. Influenza and Pneumococcal Vaccination Rates Among Persons with Diabetes
Mellitus—United States, 1997. *Morbidity and Mortality Weekly Report* 48(42):961-967.

_____. 1999b. Reasons Reported by Medicare Beneficiaries for Not Receiving Influenza and
Pneumococcal Vaccinations. *Morbidity and Mortality Weekly Report* 48(39):556-560.

_____. 2000. National, State, and Urban Area Vaccination Coverage Levels Among Children
Aged 19–35 Months—United States, 1999. *Morbidity and Mortality Weekly Report*
49(26):585-589.

_____. 2001a. *Advisory Committee on Immunization Practices (ACIP) Policies and Procedures*,
(December 28, 2001).

_____. 2001b. *ACIP Votes to Temporarily Revise Recommendations for Pneumococcal Conjugate
Vaccine (PCV-7) and Votes to Continue Previously Issued Diphtheria, Tetanus, and Pertussis
(DTaP) Recommendations*. Accessed December 7, 2003. Available at: http://
www.cdc.gov/nip/news/shortages/pneumo-and-dtap.htm.

_____. 2002a. National, State, and Urban Area Vaccination Coverage Levels Among Chil-
dren Aged 19-35 Months—United States, 2001. *Morbidity and Mortality Weekly Report*
51(3):664-666.

_____. 2002b. Deaths: Leading Causes for 2000. *National Vital Statistics Reports* 50(16).

_____. 2002c. *READII Handout*, National Partnership for Immunization Congressional Edu-
cation Session (July 31).

_____. 2002d. Influenza and Pneumococcal Vaccination Levels Among Persons Aged > 65
Years—United States, 2001. *Morbidity and Mortality Weekly Report* 51(45):1019–1024.

_____. 2002e. Email from K. Edwards, March 1. (Available from IOM.)

_____. 2002f. Data from the 2002 National Immunization Survey. Email from A. Bhatt, De-
cember 17. (Available from IOM.)

_____.2002g. Data from the 2002 National Immunization Survey. Email from L. Rodewald,
November 4. (Available from IOM.)

_____. 2002h. Data from the 2002 National Immunization Survey. Email from P. Smith, June
26. (Available from IOM.)

_____.2002i. Data from unpublished CDC report. Email from A. Bhatt, December 16. (Available from IOM.)

_____. 2002j. Vaccine Development and Testing. Vaccine Fact Sheets. Accessed July 27, 2002. Available at: www.cdc.gov/od/nvpo/fs_tableII_doc1.htm.

_____. 2002k. Vaccine Product Approval Process. Vaccine Fact Sheets. Accessed July 27, 2002. Available at: www.cdc.gov/od/nvpo/fs_tableII_doc2.htm.

_____. 2002l. Vaccine price data complied by CDC. Emails from R. Ellington between July and September 2002. (Available from IOM.)

_____. 2002m. Email from R. Ellington, July 26. (Available from IOM.)

_____. 2002n. Comments from D. O'Mara on December 1993 Abt Report Titled: Cost-Effectiveness Study of Medicare Coverage of Influenza Vaccine, July. Unpublished. (Available from IOM.)

_____. 2003a. Email from A. Bhatt, June 20, 2003. (Available from IOM.)

_____. 2003b. *Estimated Vaccination Coverage With Individual Vaccines and Selected Vaccination Series by 24 Months of Age by Immunization Action Plan Area—U.S.A., National Immunization Survey.* Accessed April 16, 2003. Available at: http://www.cdc.gov/nip/coverage/NIS/98-99/24months_urb.xls.

_____. 2003c. Email from A. Bhatt, April 4. (Available from IOM.)

_____. 2003d. *CDC Vaccine Price List.* Accessed April 1, 2003. Available at: http://www.cdc.gov/nip/vfc/cdc_vac_price_list.htm.

_____. 2003e. *Recommended Childhood Immunization Schedule, United States, 2002.* Accessed March 28, 2003. Available at: http://www.cdc.gov/nip/recs/child-schedule-twopages.pdf.

_____. 2003f. *Recommended Adult Immunization Schedule, 2002-2003.* Accessed March 28, 2003. Available at: http://www.cdc.gov/nip/recs/adult-schedule.

_____. 2003g. Email from A. Bhatt, July 10. (Available from IOM.)

_____. 2003h. *Current Vaccine Delays and Shortages.* Accessed March 28, 2003. Available at: http://www.cdc.gov/nip/news/shortages/default.htm#Which.

Clarke, B. 2002. Presentation to *Strengthening the Supply of Routinely Recommended Vaccines in the US,* the National Vaccine Advisory Committee, Washington, DC (February 11).

Cohen, J. 2002. U.S. Vaccine Supply Falls Seriously Short. *Science* 295:1998-2001.

Cohen, J.W., and P.J. Cunningham. 1995. Medicaid Physician Fee Levels and Children's Access to Care. *Health Affairs* 14(1):255-262.

Crawford, L. 2002. *FDA's Role in Maintaining the Supply of Childhood Vaccines. Testimony Before the Committee on Governmental Affairs, United States Senate* (June 12).

Darden, P., J. Taylor, and D. Brooks. 1999. Polio Immunization Practices of Pediatricians. Paper Presented Before the Pediatric Academic Societies meeting, San Diego, California.

Davidson, A., P. Melinkovich, B. Beatty, V. Chandramouli, S. Hambridge, S. Phibbs, P. Braun, C. LeBaron, and J. Steiner. 2003. Immunization Registry Accuracy: Improvement with Progressive Clinical Application. *American Journal of Preventive Medicine* 24(3):276-280.

Davis, M., J. Zimmerman, R. Wheeler, and G. Freed. 2002. Childhood Vaccine Purchase Costs in the Public Sector: Past Trends, Future Expectations. *American Journal of Public Health* 92(12):1982-1986.

DeBrock, L., and H. Grabowski. 1985. Economic Aspects of Vaccine Innovation and Manufacturing. In: *Vaccine Supply and Innovation.* Institute of Medicine. Pp. 45-64. Washington, DC: National Academy Press.

Dickey L., and D. Petitti. 1992. Patient-Held Minirecord to Promote Adult Preventive Care. *Journal of Family Practice* 34:457-463.

DiMasi, J., R. Hansen, and H. Grabowski, and L. Lasagna. 1991. Costs of Innovation in the Pharmaceutical Industry. *Journal of Health Economics* 10(2):107-142.

DiMasi, J., R. Hansen, and H. Grabowski. 2003. The Price of Innovation: New Estimates of Drug Development Costs. *Journal of Health Economics* 22(2):325-330.

Ekwueme, D., P. Strebel, S. Hadler, M. Meltzer, J. Allen, and J. Livengood. 2000. Economic Evaluation of the Use of Diphtheria, Tetanus, and Acellular Pertussis Vaccine (DTaP) or Diphtheria, Tetanus, and Whole-Cell Pertussis Vaccine (DTwP) in the United States, 1997. *Archives of Pediatric and Adolescent Medicine* 154:797-803.

Ellis, R., and G. Douglas. 1994. Combination Vaccines. *International Journal of Technology Assessment in Health Care* 10(1):185-192.

Fairbrother, G., and A. Haidery. 2002. *Vaccine Purchase and Distribution: Proposed Changes in Vaccine Supply and Delivery Policies.* Unpublished. (Available from IOM.)

Fairbrother, G., S. Friedman, K. Dumont, and K. Lobach. 1996. Markers for Primary Care: Missed Opportunities to Immunize and Screen for Lead and Tuberculosis by Private Physicians Serving Large Numbers of Inner-City Medicaid-Eligible Children. *Pediatrics* 97(6 Pt 1):785-790.

Fairbrother, G., S. Friedman, K. Hanson, and G. Butts. 1997. Effect of the Vaccines for Children Program on Inner-City Neighborhood Physicians. *Archives of Pediatric and Adolescent Medicine* 151(12):1229-1235.

Fairbrother, G., K. Hanson, S. Friedman, and G. Butts. 1999. The Impact of Physician Bonuses, Enhanced Fees, and Feedback on Childhood Immunization Coverage Rates. *American Journal of Public Health* 89(2):171-175.

Fairbrother, G., H. Kuttner, W. Miller, R. Hogan, H. McPhillips, K. Johnson, and E. Alexander. 2000. Findings from Case Studies of State and Local Immunization Programs. *American Journal of Preventive Medicine* 19(3 Supplement):54-77.

Federal Funds Information for States. 2002. *Growth in Federal Grants for Immunization, Issue Brief 02-58.* November 7, 2002.

Fee, E., and T. Brown. 2002. The Unfulfilled Promise of Public Health: Deja Vu All Over Again. *Health Affairs* 21(6):31-43.

Feikema, S., R. Klevens, M. Washington, and L. Barker. 2000. Extraimmunization Among U.S. Children. *Journal of the American Medical Association* 283(10):1311-1317.

Felton, H. 1957. Pertussis: Current Status of Prevention and Treatment. *Pediatric Clinics of North America* 31:271-283.

Fielding, J., W. Cumberland, and L. Pettitt. 1994. Immunization Status of Children of Employers in a Large Corporation. *Journal of the American Medical Association* 271:525-530.

Fine, A. 2003. *Diphtheria, Tetanus and Acellular Pertussis Vaccine (DTaP): A Case Study.* Unpublished. (Available from IOM.)

Finkelstein, A. 2003. *Health Policy and Technological Change: Evidence from the Vaccine Industry.* Working Paper 9460. Cambridge, MA: National Bureau of Economic Research.

Fontanesi, J., M. DeGuire, M. Holcomb, and M. Sawyer. 2001. The Cost to Immunize During Well-Child Visits. *American Journal of Medical Quality* 16(6):196-201.

Food and Drug Administration (FDA). 2003. *Product Approval Letter to MedImmune Vaccines, Inc.,* dated June 17, 2003. Accessed July 10, 2003. Available at: http://www.fda.gov/cber/approvltr/inflmed061703L.htm.

_____. 2002. *New Pediatric Combination Vaccine Approved. FDA Talk Paper.* Accessed December 16, 2002. Available at: http://www.fda.gov/bbs/topics/ANSWERS/2002/ANSO1181.html.

Foulkes, M., and S. Ellenberg. 2002. *Vaccine Efficacy and Safety Evaluation.* In: National Institutes of Health. *The Jordan Report.*

France, E. 2000. Vaccine Financing: The View of Managed Care. *American Journal of Preventive Medicine* 19(3 Supplement):23-25.

Freed, G., and A. Cowan. 2002. *State-Level Perspectives on Vaccine Purchase Financing.* December 2002. Unpublished. (Available from IOM.)

Freed, G., S. Clark, D. Pathman, R. Schectman, and J. Serling. 1999. Impact of North Carolina's Universal Vaccine Purchase Program by Children's Insurance Status. *Archives of Pediatric and Adolescent Medicine* 153:748-754.

Freed, G., S. Clark, and A. Cowan. 2000. State-Level Perspectives on Immunization Policies, Practices, and Program Financing in the 1990s. *American Journal of Preventive Medicine* 19(3 Supplement):32-44.

Freed, G., M. Davis, M. Andreae, S. Bass, and H. Weinblatt. 2002a. Reimbursement for Prevnar: A Modern-Day Version of Hercules and the Hydra. *Pediatrics* 110(2 Pt 1):399-400.

Freed, G., M. Andreae, A. Cowan, and S. Katz. 2002b. The Process of Public Policy Formulation: The Case of Thimerosal in Vaccines. *Pediatrics* 109(6):1153-1159.

Freeman, P., and A. Robbins. 1991. The Elusive Promise of Vaccines. *The American Prospect* 93.

Gabel, J., A. Sasso, and T. Rice. 2002. Consumer-Driven Health Plans: Are They More Than Talk Now? *Health Affairs* 21(1):W395-W407.

Gangarosa, E., A. Galazka, C. Wolfe, L. Phillips, R. Gangarosa, E. Miller, and R. Chen. 1998. Impact of Anti-Vaccine Movements on Pertussis Control: The Untold Story. *The Lancet* 351:356-361.

General Accounting Office. 1995. *Reexamination of Program Goals and Implementation Needed to Ensure Vaccination.* Washington, DC: U.S. General Accounting Office.

_____. 2001. *Health Centers and Rural Health Clinics: Payments Likely to Be Constrained Under Medicaid's New System.* Washington, DC: U.S. General Accounting Office (June).

_____. 2002. *Childhood Vaccines: Ensuring an Adequate Supply Poses Continuing Challenges.* 2002. Washington, DC: U.S. General Accounting Office.

GlaxoSmithKline. 2002. *Letter to the U.S. General Accounting Office* (April 30).

Glazner, J., J. Steiner, K. Haas, B. Renfrew, M. Deutchman, and S. Berman. 2001. Is Reimbursement for Childhood Immunizations Adequate? Evidence from Two Rural Areas in Colorado. *Public Health Reports* 116(3):219-225.

Glode, M. 2001. Combination vaccines: Practical Considerations for Public Health and Private Practice. *Pediatric Infectious Disease Journal* 20(11):S19-S22 (November).

Gold, M., L. Russel, J. Siegel, and M. Weinstein (eds.). 1996. *Cost-Effectiveness in Health and Medicine.* Oxford: Oxford University Press.

Grabowski, H., and J. Vernon. 1997. *The Search for New Vaccines: The Effects of the Vaccines for Children Program.* Washington, DC: AEI Press.

Grabowski, H., and J. Vernon. 2000. The distribution of Sales Revenue from Pharmaceutical Innovation. *PharmacoEconomics* 18(Supplement 1):21-32.

Hay, J., and D. Zammit. 2002. *Vaccine Policy Perspectives: Market Strategies.* Unpublished. (Available from IOM.)

Hirschler, B. 2002. Vaccine Renaissance Outpaces Sickly Drug Industry. *Reuters News Service,* December 5, 2002.

Horne, P., K. Saarlas, and A. Hinman. 2000. Costs of Immunization Registries: Experiences From the All Kids Count Projects. *American Journal of Preventive Medicine* 19(2):94-98.

Hughart, N., D. Strobino, E. Holt, B. Guyer, W. Hou, A. Huq, and A. Ross. 1999. The Relation of Parent and Provider Characteristics to Vaccination Status of Children in Private Practices and Managed Care Organizations in Maryland. *Medical Care* 37(1):44-55.

Huse, D., H. Meissner, M. Lacey, and G. Oster. 1994. Childhood Vaccination Against Chickenpox and Analysis of Benefits and Costs. *Journal of Pediatrics* 124:869-874.

Institute of Medicine. 1985. *Vaccine Supply and Innovation.* Washington, DC: National Academy Press.

_____. 1993. *The Children's Vaccine Initiative.* Washington, DC: National Academy Press.

_____. 1995. *The Children's Vaccine Initiative: Continuing Activities*. Washington, DC: National Academy Press.

_____. 2000a. *Calling the Shots*. Washington, DC: National Academy Press.

_____. 2000b. *Vaccines for the 21st Century: A Tool for Decisionmaking*. Washington, DC: National Academy Press.

_____. 2001. *Council of the Institute of Medicine Statement on Vaccine Development*. Washington, DC (November 5).

_____. 2002a. *Setting the Course: Part 1-Summary of the Chicago Workshop*. Washington, DC: National Academy Press.

_____. 2002b. *Setting the Course: Part 2-Summary of the Austin Workshop*. Washington, DC: National Academy Press.

_____. 2002c. *Health Insurance Is a Family Matter*. Washington, DC: The National Academies Press.

_____. 2002d. *Fostering Rapid Advances in Health Care*. Washington, DC: The National Academies Press.

_____. 2002e. *Protecting Our Forces: Improving Vaccine Acquisition and Availability in the U.S. Military*. Washington, DC: The National Academies Press.

_____. 2003a. *Setting the Course: Part 3-Summary of the Los Angeles Workshop*. Washington, DC: The National Academies Press.

_____. 2003b. *The Future of the Public's Health in the 21st Century*. Washington, DC: The National Academies Press.

Ives, D., J. Lave, N. Traven, and L. Kuller. 1994. Impact of Medicare Reimbursement on Influenza Vaccination Rates in the Elderly. *Preventive Medicine* 23(2):134-141.

Jacobs, R., and A. Meyerhoff. 2001. Comparative Cost Effectiveness of Varicella, Hepatitis A, and Pneumococcal Conjugate Vaccines. *Preventive Medicine* 33:639-645.

Johnson, A. 2002. *Presentation to the Working Group on Cell Culture-Based Influenza Vaccines* (August 14).

Johnson, K., A. Sardell, and B. Richards. 2000. Federal Immunization Policy and Funding: A History of Responding to Crises. *American Journal of Preventive Medicine* 19(3S):99-112.

Kaiser Family Foundation and Health Research and Educational Trust [KFF–HRET]. 2002. *Employer Health Benefits. 2002 Annual Survey*. Washington, DC.

Kelly, D., B. Barnow, W.Gold, and L. Aron, 1993. *An Analysis of the Federal and State Roles in the Immunization of Preschool Children*. Washington, DC: Lewin–VHI (January 18).

Kremer, M. 1998. Patent Buyouts: A Mechanism for Encouraging Innovation. *Quarterly Journal of Economics* 113(4):1137-1167.

_____. 2000a. *Creating Markets for New Vaccines. Part II: Design Issues*. Working Paper 7716. Cambridge, MA: National Bureau of Economic Research.

_____. 2000b. *Creating Markets for New Vaccines. Part I: Rationale*. Working Paper 7716. Cambridge, MA: National Bureau of Economic Research.

Ladd, H., and J. Hansen (eds.). 1999. *Making Money Matter: Financing America's Schools*. Washington, DC: National Academy Press.

Laffont, J. 1994. The New Economics of Regulation Ten Years After. *Econometrica* 623:507-537.

Lane, K. 2002. Presentation to *Strengthening the Supply of Routinely Recommended Vaccines in the US*, the National Vaccine Advisory Committee, Washington, DC (February 11).

Le, C. 2001. Combination Vaccines; Choices or Chaos? A Practitioners Perspective. *Clinical Infectious Diseases* 33(Supplement 4):S367-S371.

LeBaron, C., L. Rodewald, and S. Humiston. 1999. How Much Time Is Spent on Well-Child Care and Vaccinations?" *Archives of Pediatric and Adolescent Medicine* 153:1154-1159.

Lett, S. 2002. *Presentation to the Work Group on Public Health Options for Implementing Vaccine Recommendations Town Hall Meeting*, Boston, April 18, 2002.

Lichtenberg, F. 2002. *Trends in Vaccine Prices, 1992-2002.* Unpublished. (Available from IOM.)

Lieu, T., S. Cochi, S. Black, E. Halloran, H. Shinefield, S. Holmes, M. Wharton, and E. Washington. 1994a. Cost-Effectiveness of a Routine Varicella Vaccination Program for US Children. *Journal of the American Medical Association* 271:375-381.

Lieu, T., M. Smith, P. Newacheck, D. Langthorn, P. Venkatesh, and R. Herradora. 1994b. Health Insurance and Preventive Care Sources of Children at Public Immunization Clinics. *Pediatrics* 93(3):373-378.

Lieu, T., G. Ray, S. Black, J. Butler. J. Klein, R. Breiman, M. Miller, and H. Shinefield. 2000a. Projected Cost-Effectiveness of Pneumococcal Conjugate Vaccination of Healthy Infants and Young Children. *Journal of the American Medical Association* 283:1460-1468.

Lieu, T., S. Black, G. Ray, K. Martin, H. Shinefield, and B. Weniger. 2000b. The Hidden Costs of Infant Vaccination. *Vaccine* 19(1):33-41.

Luman, E., M. McCauley, S. Stokley, S. Chu, and L. Pickering. 2002. Timeliness of Childhood Vaccinations. *Pediatrics* 110(5):935-939.

Lumpkin, J., and M. Richards. 2002. Transforming the Public Health Information Infrastructure. *Health Affairs* 21(6):45-56.

Lurie, N., W. Manning, C. Peterson, G. Goldberg, C. Phelps, and L. Lillard. 1987. Preventive Care: Do We Practice What We Preach? *American Journal of Public Health* 77(7):801-804.

Marketletter. 2002. Double-digit Growth Rates Elude Most Blockbuster Firms, Says *Datamonitor. Marketletter* (May 27).

Marks, J., T. Halpin, J. Irvin, D. Johnson, and J. Keller. 1979. Risk Factors Associated with Failure to Receive Vaccinations. *Pediatrics* 64(3):304-309.

Mason, D. 2002. *An Update on DTaP, MMR, PCV-7, Varicella, and Other Vaccines for the U.S. Market.* Presentation to the National Vaccine Advisory Committee Meeting of October 8.

McGuire, T. 2003. Setting Prices for New Vaccines (In Advance). Unpublished. (Available through IOM.)

Mercer Management Consulting. 2002. *Lessons Learned: New Procurement Strategies for Vaccines: Final Report to the GAVI Board.*

———. 1995. *Report on the United States Vaccine Industry.* Report to the Department of Health and Human Services.

Merck. 2002. *Merck's Response to the IOM Committee.* (Email from Maggie Keane, December 6).

Meyer, J., and E. Waldman. 2002. *Under-Insured for Vaccines. Magnitude, Causes, and Consequences.* Washington, DC: New Directions for Policy.

Meyerhoff, A., B. Weniger, and R. Jacobs. 2001. Economic Value to Parents of Reducing the Pain and Emotional Distress of Childhood Vaccine Injections. *Pediatric Infectious Disease Journal* 20(11 Suppl):S57-S62.

Miller, H. 2002. An Indefensible Epidemic. *The Wall Street Journal* (19 August).

Miller, M., and A. Hinman. 1999. Cost-Benefit and Cost-Effectiveness Analysis of Vaccine Policy. In: Plotkin, S., and W. Orenstein (eds.). *Vaccines.* London: W.B. Saunders.

Mowery, D., and V. Mitchell. 1995. Improving the Reliability of the U.S. Vaccine Supply: An Evaluation of Alternatives. *Journal of Health Politics, Policy and Law* 20(4):973-1000.

Nace, N., C. Larson, T. Lester, and J. Kosinski. 1999. Perceived Barriers to Childhood Immunization: A Physician and Parent Survey in a Southeastern Urban/Rural Community. *Tennessee Medicine* 92(7):265-268.

National Association of County and City Health Officials (NACCHO). 2003. *LPHA Infrastructure: A Chartbook.* Accessed March 29, 2003. Available at: http://www.naccho.org/files/documents/chartbook_programs18-48.pdf.

National Center for Health Statistics (NCHS). 2000. Percentage of Persons Aged >18 Years Who Reported Receiving Influenza or Pneumococcal Vaccine or Tetanus Toxoid, By Age and Selected Characteristics–National Health Interview Survey, United States, 1999. Unpublished. (Available through IOM.)

National Health Policy Forum. 2001. *The Disappearing State Surpluses: How Come, How Long, and How Will They Affect Social Service Programs.* Issue Brief No. 769. Washington, DC.

National Institutes of Health (NIH). 2002. *Improved Pertussis Vaccines: Enhancing Protection. Stories of Discovery.* Accessed June 6, 2002. Available at: www.niaid.nih.gov/publications/discovery/pertus.html.

National Vaccine Advisory Committee (NVAC). 1999. *Development of Community- and State-Based Immunization Registries,* January 12, 1999.

_____. 2003. *Strengthening the Supply of Routinely Recommended Vaccines in the United States: A Report of the National Vaccine Advisory Committee* (January).

Nexoe, J., Kragstrup, J., and T. Ronne. 1997. The Impact of Postal Invitations and User Fee on Influenza Vaccination Rates Among the Elderly: A Randomized Controlled Trial in General Practice. *Scandinavian Journal of Primary Health Care* 15:109-112.

Noble, G., R. Bernier, E. Esber, C. Hardegree, A. Hinman, D. Klein, and A. Saah. 1987. Acellular and Whole-Cell Pertussis Vaccines in Japan: Report of a Visit by US Scientists. *Journal of the American Medical Association* 257(10):1351-1356.

Ohmit S., A. Furumoto–Dawson, A. Monto, and N. Fasano. 1995. Influenza Vaccine Use among an Elderly Population in a Community Intervention. *American Journal of Preventive Medicine* 11(4):271-276.

Oram R., R. Daum, J. Seal, and D. Lauderdale, 2001. Impact of Recommendations to Suspend the Birth Dose of Hepatitis B Virus Vaccine. *Journal of the American Medical Association* 285(14):1874-1879.

Orenstein, W. 2002a. *Protecting Our Kids: What is Causing the Current Shortage in Childhood Vaccines?* Testimony to the Senate Committee on Governmental Affairs (June 6).

_____. 2002b. *Vaccine Supply-CDC Concerns.* Presentation to *Strengthening the Supply of Routinely Recommended Vaccines in the US,* the National Vaccine Advisory Committee, Washington, DC, February 11, 2002.

Orenstein, W., A. Hinman, and L. Rodewald. 1999. Public Health Considerations-United States. In: Plotkin, S., and W. Orenstein (eds.). *Vaccines.* London: W.B. Saunders.

Ortega, A., D. Stewart, S. Dowshen, and S. Katz. 2000. The Impact of a Pediatric Medical Home on Immunization Coverage. *Clinical Pediatrics* 39(2):89-96.

Pauly, M., and B. Cleff. 1995. The Economics of Vaccine Policy: An Overview of the Issues. In: *Supplying Vaccines: An Economic Analysis of Critical Issues.* Pauly, M., C. Robinson, S. Sepe, M. Sing, and M. Willian (eds.). London: IOS Press.

Pellissier, J., P. Coplan, L. Jackson, and J. May. 2000. The Effect of Additional Shots on the Vaccine Administration Process: Results of a Time-Motion Study in 2 Settings. *American Journal of Managed Care* 6(9):1038-1044.

Pisano, W. 2002. *Strengthening the Supply of Routinely Recommended Vaccines in the US.* Presentation to the National Vaccine Advisory Committee (February 11-12).

Pleis, J., and J. Gentleman. 2002. Using the National Health Interview Survey: Time Trends in Influenza Vaccination Among Targeted Adults. *Effective Clinical Practice* 5(3 Suppl):E3.

Preblud, S., W. Orenstein, J. Koplin, K. Bart, and A. Hinman. 1986. A Benefit-Cost Analysis of a Childhood Varicella Vaccination Programme. *Postgraduate Medicine Journal* 61:17-22.

Rappuoli, R., H. Miller, and S. Faldow. 2002. The Intangible Value of Vaccination. *Science* 297:937-939.

Rask, K., K. Wells, S. Kohler, C. Rust, and C. Cangialose. 2000. The Cost to Providers of Participating in an Immunization Registry. *American Journal of Preventive Medicine* 19(2):99-103.

Robinson, J. 2002. Renewed Emphasis on Consumer Cost Sharing on Health Insurance Benefit Design. *Health Affairs* 21(3):W139-W154.

Rodewald L., P. Szilagyi, J. Holl, L. Shone, J. Zwanziger, and R. Raubertas. 1997. Health Insurance for Low-Income Working Families. Effect on the Provision of Immunizations to Preschool-Age Children. *Archives of Pediatric and Adolescent Medicine* 151(8):798-803.

Rogerson, W. 1994. Economic Incentives and the Defense Procurement Process. *Journal of Economic Perspectives* 8(4):65-90.

Ruch-Ross, H., and K. O'Connor. 1994. Immunization Referral Practices of Pediatricians in the United States. *Pediatrics* 94(4 Pt 1):508-513.

Santoli, J., P. Szilagyi, and L. Rodewald. 1998. Barriers to Immunization and Missed Opportunities. *Pediatric Annals* 27(6):366-374.

Satterthwaite, P. 1997. A Randomized Intervention Study to Examine the Effect on Immunization Coverage of Making Influenza Vaccine Available at No Cost. *New Zealand Medical Journal* 110(1038):58-60.

Scherer, F. 2001. The Link Between Gross Profitability and Pharmaceutical R&D Spending. *Health Affairs* September/October:216–220.

Schulte, J., G. Bown, M. Zetzman, B. Schwartz, H. Green, C. Haley, and R. Anderson. 1991. Changing Immunization Referral Patterns Among Pediatricians, Dallas County, Texas, 1988. *Pediatrics* 87(2):204-207.

Schultz, J. 2003. Success of Vaccine Offers Promise of Cervical Cancer Prevention. *Journal of the National Cancer Institute* 95(2):102-104.

Schwartz, B., and W. Orenstein. 2001. Vaccination Policies and Programs: The Federal Government's Role in Making the System Work. *Primary Care* 28(4):697-711.

Shalala, D. 1993. *Testimony to the Joint Hearing Before the Senate Committee on Labor and Human Resources and the House Subcommittee on Health and the Environment of the Committee on Energy and Commerce* (April 21).

Sing, M., and M. Willian. 1996. Supplying Vaccines: An Overview of the Market and Regulatory Context. In: Pauly, M., C. Robinson, S. Sepe, M. Sing, and M. Willian (eds.). *Supplying Vaccines: An Economic Analysis of Critical Issues.* London: IOS Press.

SmithKline Beecham. 2000. *Development of DTaP-based Hib conjugate combination vaccines: SmithKline Beecham presentation to Vaccines and Related Biological Products Advisory Committee,* CBER, FDA (January 27).

St. Peter, R., P. Newacheck, and N. Halfon. 1992. Access to Care for Poor Children: Separate and Unequal? *Journal of the American Medical Association* 267:2760-2764.

Stille, C., and J. Christison-Lagay. 2000. Determining Immunization Rates for Inner-City Infants: Statewide Registry Data vs. Medical Record Review. *American Journal of Public Health* 90(10):1613-1615.

Stokely, S., L. Rodewald, and E. Maes. 2001. The Impact of Record Scattering on the Measurement of Immunization Coverage. *Pediatrics* 107(1):91-96.

Swartz, K. 2003. *How Insurance Companies and Health Plans Are Planning for New Vaccines.* Unpublished. (Available from IOM.)

Szilagyi, P., and L. Rodewald. 1996. Missed Opportunities for Immunizations: A Review of the Evidence. *Journal of Public Health Management Practice* 2(1):18-25.

Szilagyi, P., S. Huniston, L. Shone, M. Kolasa, and L. Rodewald. 2000a. Decline in Physician Referrals to Health Department Clinics for Immunizations: The Role of Vaccine Financing. *American Journal of Preventive Medicine* 18(4):318-324.

Szilagyi, P., S. Humiston, L. Shone, R. Barth, M. Kolasa, and L. Rodewald. 2000b. Impact of Vaccine Financing on Vaccinations Delivered by Health Department Clinics. *American Journal of Public Health* 90(5):739-745.

Tatande, M., V. Dietz, M. Lewin, and E. Zell. 1996. Health Care Characteristics and Their Association with the Vaccination Status of Children. *Archives of Pediatric and Adolescent Medicine* 150(Supple 4):abstract 161.

Taylor, J., P. Darden, E. Slora, C. Hasemeier, L. Asmussen, and R. Wasserman. 1997. The Influence of Provider Behavior, Parental Characteristics, and a Public Policy Initiative on the Immunization Status of Children Followed by Private Pediatricians: A Study from Pediatric Research in Office Settings. *Pediatrics* 99(2):209-215.

Thompson, W., D. Shay, E. Weintraub, L. Brammer, N. Cox, L. Anderson, and K. Fukuda. 2003. Mortality Associated with Influenza and Respiratory Syncytial Virus in the United States. *Journal of the American Medical Association* 289(2):179-186.

Tufts Center for the Study of Drug Development. 2001. Tufts Center for the Study of Drug Development Pegs Cost of a New Prescription Medicine at $802 Million. Press Release (November 30).

UnitedHealthcare. 2002. UnitedHealthcare. *Letter from C. Lund to G. Martens, State of Connecticut* (July 2).

U.S. Census Bureau. 2002. Health Insurance Coverage: 2001. Current Population Reports. Washington, DC: U.S. Census Bureau (September).

U.S. Department of Health and Human Services. 2000. *Healthy People 2010.* Washington, DC.
_____. 2003. *President to Propose Improvements in Childhood Vaccine Programs.* Press Release (January 25).

Wendland-Bowyer, W., and E. Askari. 2002. Vaccine Rule Could Hurt Kids: Public Health Agencies Can Turn Away the Insured. *Detroit Free Press* (July 1).

Wood, D. 2003. *Estimating Need for Publicly Purchased Vaccine for Adults and Children.* Unpublished. (Available from IOM.)

Wood, D., and N. Halfon. 1996. The Impact of the Vaccine for Children's Program on Child Immunization Delivery. A Policy Analysis. *Archives of Pediatric and Adolescent Medicine* 150(6):577-581.

Wyeth Pharmaceuticals. 2002. Wyeth Ceases Production of Its Injectable Influenza Vaccine and Pneumococcal Polysaccharide Vaccine. Press Release (November 19, 2002).

Zhou, F., K. Bisgard, H. Yusuf, R. Deuson, S. Bath, and T. Murphy. 2002. Impact of Universal *Haemophilus influenzae* Type b Vaccination Starting at 2 Months of Age in the United States: An Economic Analysis. *Pediatrics* 110(4):653-661 (October).

Zhou, F., S. Reef, M. Massoudi, M. Papania, H. Yusuf, B. Bardenheier, L. Zimmerman, and M. McCauley. In press. An Economic Analysis of the Current Universal 2-Dose MMR Vaccination Program in the United States.

Zimmerman, R., A. Medsger, E. Ricci, M. Raymund, T. Mieczkowski, and S. Grufferman. 1997. Impact of Free Vaccine and Insurance Status on Physician Referral of Children to Public Vaccine Clinics. *Journal of the American Medical Association* 278(12):996-1000.

Zimmerman, R., T. Mieczkowski, and M. Michel. 1999. Are Vaccination Rates Higher If Providers Receive Free Vaccines and Follow Contraindication Guidelines? *Family Medicine* 31(5):317-323.

Zimmerman, R., S. Van Cleve, A. Medsger, R. Mahlon, and J. Ball. 2000. Does the Vaccines for Children Program Influence Pediatric Nurse Practitioner Referral of Disadvantaged Children to Public Vaccine Clinics? *Maternal and Child Health Journal* 4(1):53-58.

Zimmerman, R., T. Mieczkowski, H. Mainzer, A. Medsger, R. Mahlon, J. Ball, and I. Jewell. 2001. Effect of the Vaccines for Children Program on Physician Referral of Children to Public Vaccine Clinics: A Pre–Post Comparison. *Pediatrics* 108(2):297-304.

Glossary

Advisory Committee on Immunization Practices (ACIP). A 15-member expert advisory body appointed by the Secretary of the U.S. Department of Health and Human Services (DHHS) to advise the Secretary and the Centers for Disease Control and Prevention (CDC) on prevention of vaccine-preventable diseases. ACIP recommends vaccines for use by the general population or targeted groups and recommends vaccines for inclusion in the Vaccines for Children (VFC) entitlement program.

Antigen. Any foreign substance in the body that triggers an immune response. A vaccine is made up of one or more antigens that trigger the body's immunity to the intended disease.

Block grant. A block grant is a federal program financing mechanism by which programmatic funds are distributed to the states, which then have considerable leeway in how they use the funds to achieve the programmatic goals. Examples of block grant programs are the Temporary Assistance for Needy Families and Maternal and Child Health grant programs.

Combination vaccine. Two or more vaccines administered in a single injection; DTaP is an example.

Community health center (CHC). CHCs are nonprofit health clinics that provide primary medical care to underserved populations. They include health centers that do and do not receive Section 330 grants from the Bureau of Primary Health Care. In 1992, an alternative term—federally qualified health center (FQHC)—was introduced to denote CHCs eligible to receive Medicare payment.

Concentration. The market shares of the largest firms indicate the concentration of the industry. Indicators of concentration include the cumulative four-firm and eight-firm market shares, as well as the Herfindahl Index, which is calculated as the sum of the squared market shares of all of the individual firms.

Copayment. A fixed amount of money paid by an insurance beneficiary at the time of service. Typically ranging from $5 to $25, this form of patient cost sharing is designed to provide an incentive for the patient to utilize health resources wisely.

Cost sharing. A health insurance provision that requires the insured individual to pay some portion of medical expenses through three usual methods—copayments, coinsurance, and deductibles.

Coverage. In the public health literature, usually refers to the rate of immunization of a population; in the economic and health policy literature, usually means enrollment in a health insurance plan. To avoid confusion, the term is used exclusively in this report to mean insurance coverage.

Crowd-out. The tendency of public programs to absorb some proportion of individuals or entities that would otherwise participate in private markets. In health insurance markets, the term commonly refers to the phenomenon whereby privately insured individuals or companies drop private health insurance coverage and take advantage of a public program.

Current Good Manufacturing Practices. FDA standards for vaccine manufacturing processes and facilities; must be met before and during production of vaccines.

Deductible. A preset amount below which insurance policies typically do not pay for expenses. Once the deductible has been satisfied, all other expenses are paid according to the terms of the policy.

Defined contribution plan. Also known as a consumer-driven health plan, a group health insurance program that provides employees with health spending accounts with which they can purchase a high-deductible insurance policy; pay for cost sharing; and purchase extended benefits, such as a fitness center membership. Once all the money in the account has been used, employees must pay for any copayments and other noncatastrophic care out of pocket. It is called a defined contribution plan because the employer contributes a predefined amount; the benefits received by the employee vary according to his or her medical experience and personal choices. The typical employee benefit plan, in contrast, is a defined benefit policy because the benefits that can be received by the employee are defined, and the amount paid by the employer varies according to the employee's utilization of medical services.

DTP/DTaP. A combination vaccine that immunizes against diptheria, a respiratory disease; tetanus, a disease of the nervous system contracted from the environment; and pertussis, also known as whooping cough. All three can be fatal. DTaP includes the newer "acelullar" version of the pertussis antigen, which does not contain whole cells.

Eligibility. Criteria that establish whether an individual is qualified to participate in a particular program. For example, federally defined eligibility for participation in the VFC program requires that an individual be between the ages of 0 and 18 and fall into one of the following categories: Medicaid-eligible, uninsured, Native American, Alaskan Native, or underinsured and receiving vaccination at an FQHC.

ERISA. The Employee Retirement Income Security Act, a federal law passed in 1974 that established standards, reporting, and disclosure requirements for employer-funded pension and health benefit programs. By preempting state law, self-funded health benefit programs are exempted from state insurance regulation.

Externality, positive consumption, or spillover effect. When a consumption of a product by one person benefits others, the benefit to others is a positive consumption externality or spillover effect. For example, the measles vaccine protects not just the individual being immunized but the community at large by establishing herd immunity.

Federally qualified health center (FQHC). A community health center that is eligible to receive Medicare payment.

Fee, administration. The payment or fee to a clinician or provider organization for the administration of a vaccine, exclusive of the reimbursement for the cost of the vaccine itself.

Fragmentation. A term used throughout this report to refer broadly to adverse consequences of multiple funding sources and multiple providers for immunization. Such consequences include difficulties in determining patient eligibility because of multiple funding programs, increases in referrals from the private to the public sector, and scattering of medical records among multiple providers.

Health maintenance organization (HMO). An entity that provides both insurance and medical services to members, who pay a fixed premium in advance without regard to the actual services used. Members must use selected providers that are affiliated with the HMO or pay extra and must abide by certain restrictions in their utilization of services.

Health plan/health insurance plan. In this report, both terms refer to health insurance companies and the specified services provided to insured individuals under the terms of the plan. In this context, "health plan" does not imply an HMO or other type of managed care.

Herd immunity. Immunity among a large percentage of a population, which protects even those not immunized by interrupting the transmission of disease.

Hib. *Haemophilus influenzae* type B, a bacterial disease that is responsible for meningitits, pneumonia, and other diseases. Also denotes the vaccine that protects against it.

Hepatitis A. A serious viral infection. Hep A is often used to indicate the vaccine that protects against it.

Hepatitis B. A dangerous viral disease that affects the liver. Hep B and HBV are often used to indicate the vaccine that protects against it.

Immunization. The process by which a person or animal becomes protected by a vaccine against a disease. Interchangeable with "vaccination" or "inoculation."

Influenza. A seasonal, respiratory virus commonly known as the flu.

IPV. Inactivated poliovirus vaccine (see **poliomyelitis**).

Market power. The ability of an entity to negotiate more favorable prices or other terms based on its large percentage share of a market. Monopolies and monopsonies have the maximum market power over their respective product and input markets. Market power is correlated with the degree of industry **concentration** (see definition above).

Meningococcal vaccine. A vaccine that protects against *neisseria meningitidis,* a bacterial infection that is the leading cause of bacterial meningitis and sepsis in children and young adults. The disease is fatal for about 10 percent of those who contract it.

MMR. A combination vaccine that immunizes against measles, a serious respiratory virus; mumps, a viral disease that that can cause deafness; and rubella, a mild rash with sometimes serious complications, also known as German measles.

Monopsony. A market characterized by a single buyer. A monopsonistic market behaves like a monopsony by virtue of having a very dominant buyer.

National immunization system. The constellation of private and public programs, services, providers, and public health activities that finance, deliver, promote, and monitor immunization services and outcomes.

National Vaccine Advisory Committee. An advisory group that makes recommendations to the National Vaccine Program Office (see below) regarding national immunization policy and strategies.

National Vaccine Program Office. The office within DHHS that is responsible for coordinating national immunization efforts across multiple agencies.

OPV. Oral poliovirus vaccine (see **poliomyelitis**).

Out-of-pocket expenses. In health insurance, medical or related expenses that must be paid by the patient under the terms of the insurance contract. Includes copayments (or copays), coinsurance, and deductibles. Also known as cost sharing (see definition above).

Pneumococcal conjugate vaccine (PCV-7). Vaccine that protects against *streptococcus pneumoniae* bacteria, a leading cause of severe respiratory and ear infections in children. A conjugate vaccine joins together two compounds, usually a protein and a polysaccharide, to enhance a vaccine's potency. Also, this vaccine is 7 valent, meaning that it contains antigens from seven different disease-causing agents.

Pneumococcal polysaccharide vaccine (PPV). Vaccine, primarily for adults, that protects against *streptococcus pneumoniae* bacteria, a leading cause of pneumonia, bacteremia, and meningitis. A polysaccharide is a vaccine containing multiple chains of sugars that resemble the surface of the bacteria.

Poliomyelitis (also **polio**). An infectious viral disease that attacks the nervous system and can cause paralysis and death. OPV is the oral poliovirus vaccine that protects against the disease; IPV is the currently recommended, inactivated (or killed organism) version.

Preferred provider organization (PPO). An insurance entity through which members receive services from a network of providers at one cost-sharing level, or from non-network providers at a higher level of cost sharing. It is generally less restrictive than an HMO.

Provider. In this report, refers to both a medical professional and an institution engaged in patient care, such as a physician, a nurse, a hospital, or a clinic.

Public good. A product whose benefits may be provided to all people at no greater cost than that to provide it to one person. The benefits of the product are indivisible, and people cannot be excluded from using it. For example, national defense is considered a public good because it benefits everyone and can exclude no one. In this way, a public good contrasts with a private good, such as bread, which if consumed by one person cannot be consumed by another.

Public health clinic. In this report, denotes any publicly funded medical clinic, including community health centers, rural health centers, local health department clinics, and federally qualified health centers.

Recommended vaccine. A vaccine that has been recommended by ACIP for universal use or use among target populations based on the vaccine's efficacy, safety, and indications. Recommended vaccines are listed on CDC's childhood or adult vaccine schedule.

Schedule, immunization or vaccine. See **recommended vaccines**.

Section 317. Section 317 of the Public Health Services Act, enacted in 1963, established a national program of funding to states for the purchase of vaccines and for investments in immunization infrastructure.

Societal benefit. The total benefits of a vaccine, including both the private benefits to the person receiving it and the public benefits to others. Using this approach, a monetary value is assigned to all benefits associated with a new vaccine that can be determined and measured (for example, future medical costs that are averted, as well as additional life-years and enhanced quality of life). The sum of these values represents the vaccine's societal benefit. This calculation involves certain technical challenges and requires a consistent methodology and set of assumptions for all vaccines.

Spillover effect. See **externality**.

Tetanus. An often fatal bacterial infection transmitted through open wounds. Tetanus toxoid (TT) is the vaccine that protects against tetanus. Tetanus toxoid is commonly combined with other antigens to create combination vaccine products, pediatric DT or adult Td (tetanus-diphtheria) and DTaP (diphtheria-tetanus-acellular pertussis).

Thimerosal. An ethyl mercury-containing preservative used in vaccines that enabled multiple vaccinations from a single vial. Recently, the FDA required the removal of thimerosal from all recommended vaccines.

Universal purchase. Refers to government purchasing of all vaccines for all or most of the population, regardless of private insurance coverage. Some states currently have universal purchase programs.

Vaccination. The process by which a person or animal becomes protected by a vaccine against a disease. Interchangeable with "immunization" or "inoculation."

Vaccine Adverse Events Reporting System (VAERS). A system for tracking data on adverse side effects from vaccination.

Vaccine Injury Compensation Program (VICP). A program established by the National Vaccine Injury Compensation Act to provide assistance to those suffering serious adverse events as a result of routine vaccination. Designed to protect vaccine companies from product liability lawsuits from rare events.

Vaccine pipeline. The collection of vaccines in various stages of active research and development that are considered likely candidates to become available in the foreseeable future.

Vaccine schedule. A table identifying vaccines, their doses, and the timing of their administration as recommended by ACIP.

Vaccines for Children (VFC) Program. Enacted in 1993 and implemented in 1994. VFC is a federal entitlement program that provides recommended childhood vaccines to children between the ages of 0 and 18 in the following categories: Medicaid-eligible, uninsured, Native American, Alaska Native, or receiving vaccination at a federally qualified health center.

Varicella. Chickenpox, a viral infection causing red blotches on the skin. Also, the vaccine that protects against it.

Appendix A

Recommended Vaccine Schedules (Childhood and Adult)

This appendix includes reprints of the CDC recommended immunization schedule for children, adults, and adults with medical conditions. The figures have been reprinted from the following sources:

- Figure A-1: Recommended Adult Immunization Schedule, United States, 2002–2003.
  Source: www.cdc.gov/mmwr/preview/mmwrhtml/mm5140a5. htm.
- Figure A-2: Recommended Immunizations for Adults with Medical Conditions, United States, 2002-2003.
  Source: www.cdc..gov/mmwr/preview/mmwrhtml/mm5140a5.htm.
- Figure A-3: Recommended Childhood Immunization Schedule, United States, 2002.
  Source: www.cdc.gov/nip/recs/child-schedule.htm.

Recommended Adult Immunization Schedule — UNITED STATES · 2002-2003

Legend
For all persons in this group
Catch-up on childhood vaccinations
For persons with medical/exposure indications

VACCINE / AGE	19-49 YEARS	50-64 YEARS	65 YEARS & OLDER
Tetanus, Diphtheria (Td)*	1 dose booster every 10 years		
Influenza	1 dose annually for persons with medical or occupational indications, or household contacts of persons with indications	1 annual dose	
Pneumococcal (polysaccharide)	1 dose for persons with medical or other indications. (1 dose revaccination for immunosuppressive conditions)		1 dose for unvaccinated persons / 1 dose revaccination
Hepatitis B*	3 doses (0, 1-2, 4-6 months) for persons with medical, behavioral, occupational, or other indications		
Hepatitis A	2 doses (0, 6-12 months) for persons with medical, behavioral, occupational, or other indications		
Measles, Mumps, Rubella (MMR)*	1 dose if measles, mumps or rubella vaccination history is unreliable; 2 doses for persons with occupational or other indications		
Varicella*	2 doses (0, 4-8 weeks) for persons who are susceptible		
Meningococcal (polysaccharide)	1 dose for persons with medical or other indications		

* Covered by the Vaccine Injury Compensation Program. For information on how to file a claim, call **1-800-338-2382**. Please also visit **www.hrsa.osp.gov/vicp.** To file a claim for vaccine injury, write: U.S. Court of Federal Claims, 717 Madison Place, NW, Washington, DC 20005. Telephone 202-219-9657.

This schedule indicates the recommended age groups for routine administration of currently licensed vaccines for persons 19 years of age and older. Licensed combination vaccines may be used whenever any components of the combination are indicated and the vaccine's other components are not contraindicated. Providers should consult the manufacturers' package inserts for detailed recommendations.

APPROVED BY THE ADVISORY COMMITTEE ON IMMUNIZATION PRACTICES (ACIP) AND
ACCEPTED BY THE AMERICAN COLLEGE OF OBSTETRICIANS AND GYNECOLOGISTS (ACOG)
AND THE AMERICAN ACADEMY OF FAMILY PHYSICIANS (AAFP)

CDC National Immunization Hotline:
800-232-2522 ENGLISH · 800-232-0233 ESPAÑOL

Report all clinically significant post-vaccination reactions to the Vaccine Adverse Event Reporting System (VAERS). Reporting forms and instructions on filing a VAERS report are available by calling **1-800-822-7967** or from the VAERS website at **www.vaers.org.**

For additional information about the vaccines listed above and contraindications for immunization, please visit the National Immunization Program Website at **www.cdc.gov/nip** or call the National Immunization Hotline, **1-800-232-2522** (English) or **1-800-232-0233** (Spanish).

FIGURE A-1 Recommended Adult Immunization Schedule, United States, 2002-2003.

Recommended Immunizations for Adults with Medical Conditions

UNITED STATES • 2002-2003

Legend: ▇ For all persons in this group ▇ Catch-up on childhood vaccinations ▇ For persons with medical/exposure indications ▇ Contraindicated

Medical Conditions ▼ / Vaccine ▶	Tetanus-Diphtheria (Td)*	Influenza	Pneumococcal (polysaccharide)	Hepatitis B*	Hepatitis A	Measles, Mumps, Rubella (MMR)*	Varicella*
Pregnancy		A					
Diabetes, Heart Disease, Chronic Pulmonary Disease, Chronic Liver Disease, including Chronic Alcoholism		B	C		D		
Congenital Immunodeficiency, Leukemia, Lymphoma, Generalized Malignancy, Therapy with Alkylating Agents, Antimetabolites, Radiation or Large Amounts of Corticosteroids			E				F
Renal Failure/End Stage Renal Disease, Recipients of Hemodialysis or Clotting Factor Concentrates			E	G			
Asplenia, including Elective Splenectomy and Terminal Complement Component Deficiencies			E, H, I				
HIV Infection			E, J			K	

* Covered by the Vaccine Injury Compensation Program.

A. If pregnancy is at second or third trimester during influenza season.

B. Although chronic liver disease and alcoholism are not indicator conditions for influenza vaccination, give one dose annually if the patient is 50 years or older, has other indications for influenza vaccine, or if patient requests vaccination.

C. Asthma is an indicator condition for influenza but not for pneumococcal vaccination.

D. For all persons with chronic liver disease.

E. Revaccinate once after five years or more have elapsed since initial vaccination.

F. Persons with impaired humoral but not cellular immunity may be vaccinated. *MMWR* 1999;48 (RR-06):1-5.

G. Hemodialysis patients: Use special formulation of vaccine (40 ug/mL) or two 1.0 mL 20 ug doses given at one site. Vaccinate early in the course of renal disease. Assess antibody titers to hep B surface antigen (anti-HBs) levels annually. Administer additional doses if anti-HBs levels decline to <10 milli international units (mIU)/mL.

H. Also administer meningococcal vaccine.

I. Elective splenectomy: vaccinate at least two weeks before surgery.

J. Vaccinate as close to diagnosis as possible when CD4 cell counts are highest.

K. Withhold MMR or other measles-containing vaccines from HIV-infected persons with evidence of severe immunosuppression. *MMWR* 1996; 45:603-606, *MMWR* 1992; 41 (RR-17):1-19

FIGURE A-2 Recommended Immunizations for Adults with Medical Conditions, United States, 2002-2003.

Recommended Childhood Immunization Schedule
United States, 2002

range of recommended ages | catch-up vaccination | preadolescent assessment

Vaccine ▲ / Age ▶	Birth	1 mo	2 mos	4 mos	6 mos	12 mos	15 mos	18 mos	24 mos	4-6 yrs	11-12 yrs	13-18 yrs
Hepatitis B[1]	Hep B #1	Hep B #2 (only if mother HBsAg (-))			Hep B #3						Hep B series	
Diphtheria, Tetanus, Pertussis[2]			DTaP	DTaP	DTaP		DTaP	DTaP		DTaP	Td	
Haemophilus influenzae Type b[3]			Hib	Hib	Hib	Hib						
Inactivated Polio[4]			IPV	IPV	IPV	IPV				IPV		
Measles, Mumps, Rubella[5]						MMR #1				MMR #2		MMR #2
Varicella[6]						Varicella				Varicella		
Pneumococcal[7]			PCV	PCV	PCV	PCV	PCV			PCV	PPV	
Hepatitis A[8]									Hepatitis A series			
Influenza[9]						Influenza (yearly)						

---- Vaccines below this line are for selected populations ----

This schedule indicates the recommended ages for routine administration of currently licensed childhood vaccines, as of December 1, 2001, for children through age 18 years. Any dose not given at the recommended age should be given at any subsequent visit when indicated and feasible. ■ Indicates age groups that warrant special effort to administer those vaccines not previously given. Additional vaccines may be licensed and recommended during the year. Licensed combination vaccines may be used whenever any components of the combination are indicated and the vaccine's other components are not contraindicated. Providers should consult the manufacturers' package inserts for detailed recommendations.

Approved by the Advisory Committee on Immunization Practices (www.cdc.gov/nip/acip) the American Academy of Pediatrics (www.aap.org), and the American Academy of Family Physicians (www.aafp.org).

Footnotes: Recommended Childhood Immunization Schedule
United States, 2002

1. Hepatitis B vaccine (Hep B). All infants should receive the first dose of hepatitis B vaccine soon after birth and before hospital discharge; the first dose may also be given by age 2 months if the infant's mother is HBsAg-negative. Only monovalent hepatitis B vaccine can be used for the birth dose. Monovalent or combination vaccine containing Hep B may be used to complete the series; four doses of vaccine may be administered if combination vaccine is used. The second dose should be given at least 4 weeks after the first dose, except for Hib-containing vaccine which cannot be administered before age 6 weeks. The third dose should be given at least 16 weeks after the first dose and at least 8 weeks after the second dose. The last dose in the vaccination series (third or fourth dose) should not be administered before age 6 months.

Infants born to HBsAg-positive mothers should receive hepatitis B vaccine and 0.5 mL hepatitis B immune globulin (HBIG) within 12 hours of birth at separate sites. The second dose is recommended at age 1-2 months and the vaccination series should be completed (third or fourth dose) at age 6 months.

Infants born to mothers whose HBsAg status is unknown should receive the first dose of the hepatitis B vaccine series within 12 hours of birth. Maternal blood should be drawn at the time of delivery to determine the mother's HBsAg status; if the HBsAg test is positive, the infant should receive HBIG as soon as possible (no later than age 1 week).

2. Diphtheria and tetanus toxoids and acellular pertussis vaccine (DTaP). The fourth dose of DTaP may be administered as early as age 12 months, provided 6 months have elapsed since the third dose and the child is unlikely to return at age 15-18 months. **Tetanus and diphtheria toxoids (Td)** is recommended at age 11-12 years if at least 5 years have elapsed since the last dose of tetanus and diphtheria toxoid-containing vaccine. Subsequent routine Td boosters are recommended every 10 years.

3. _Haemophilus influenzae_ type b (Hib) conjugate vaccine. Three Hib conjugate vaccines are licensed for infant use. If PRP-OMP (PedvaxHIB® or ComVax® [Merck]) is administered at ages 2 and 4 months, a dose at age 6 months is not required. DTaP/Hib combination products should not be used for primary immunization in infants at age 2, 4 or 6 months, but can be used as boosters following any Hib vaccine.

4. Inactivated poliovirus vaccine (IPV). An all-IPV schedule is recommended for routine childhood poliovirus vaccination in the United States. All children should receive four doses of IPV at age 2 months, 4 months, 6-18 months, and 4-6 years.

5. Measles, mumps, and rubella vaccine (MMR). The second dose of MMR is recommended routinely at age 4-6 years but may be administered during any visit, provided at least 4 weeks have elapsed since the first dose and that both doses are administered beginning at or after age 12 months. Those who have not previously received the second dose should complete the schedule by the visit at age 11-12 years.

6. Varicella vaccine. Varicella vaccine is recommended at any visit at or after age 12 months for susceptible children (i.e. those who lack a reliable history of chickenpox). Susceptible persons aged ≥ 13 years should receive two doses, given at least 4 weeks apart.

7. Pneumococcal vaccine. The heptavalent **pneumococcal conjugate vaccine (PCV)** is recommended for all children aged 2-23 months and for certain children aged 24-59 months. **Pneumococcal polysaccharide vaccine (PPV)** is recommended in addition to PCV for certain high-risk groups. See M M W R 2000;49(RR-9);1-37.

8. Hepatitis A vaccine. Hepatitis A vaccine is recommended for use in selected states and regions, and for certain high-risk groups; consult your local public health authority. See M M W R 1999;48(RR-12);1-37.

9. Influenza vaccine. Influenza vaccine is recommended annually for children age ≥ 6 months with certain risk factors (including but not limited to asthma, cardiac disease, sickle cell disease, HIV and diabetes; see M M W R 2001;50(RR-4);1-44), and can be administered to all others wishing to obtain immunity. Children aged ≤12 years should receive vaccine in a dosage appropriate for their age (0.25 mL if age 6-35 months or 0.5 mL if aged ≥ 3 years). Children aged ≤ 8 years who are receiving influenza vaccine for the first time should receive two doses separated by at least 4 weeks.

Additional information about vaccines, vaccine supply, and contraindications for immunization, is available at www.cdc.gov/nip or at the National Immunization Hotline, 800-232-2522 (English) or 800-232-0233 (Spanish).

FIGURE A-3 Recommended Childhood Immunization Schedule, United States, 2002.

Appendix B

List of Contributors

CENTERS FOR DISEASE CONTROL AND PREVENTION
NATIONAL IMMUNIZATION PROGRAM

Walter Orenstein, Director
Lance Rodewald, Associate Director for Science
Martin Landry, Associate Director, Planning, Evaluation and Legislation
Bill Gallo, Associate Director, Policy Planning and Legislation
Achal Bhatt, Program Officer

Lawrence Barker, Assessment Branch
Mary Ann Bryant, Contracting Officer
Margaret Coleman, Economist
K.C. Edwards, Program Officer
Rex Ellington, Technical Project Officer
Lisa Galloway, National Immunization Program
Alison Johnson, Deputy Director, Immunization Services Division
Laurie Johnson, Deputy Director, Epidemiology and Surveillance
    Division
Sharon Katz, Acting Director, Office of Program Planning and
    Evaluation
Glen Koops, Branch Chief, Program Operations
Kimberly Lane, Deputy Associate Director, Management and
    Operations
Robert Linkins, Chief, Systems Development Branch

Dean Mason, Chief, Program Support Branch, Immunization Services
    Division
Dennis O'Mara, Associate Director for Adult Immunization
Abigail Shefer, Chief, Health Services Research and Evaluation Branch
Philip Smith, National Immunization Program
Michael Washington, Industrial Engineer, Data Management Division
Bruce Weniger, Assistant Chief for Vaccine Development
Melinda Wharton, Director, Epidemiology and Surveillance Division

OTHER CONTRIBUTORS

Mohammad Akhter, American Public Health Association
Bud Anthony, Great Falls, VA
Harris Berman, Tufts Health Plan
Carmella Bocchino, American Association of Health Plans
Damian Braga, Aventis Pasteur
Kristin Butterfield, American Academy of Pediatrics
Boyd Clarke, Neose Technologies
Martha Cook, American Academy of Pediatrics
Charles Cutler, American Association of Health Plans
Jean Davis, Director, American Academy of Pediatrics
Henry Desmarais, Health Insurance Association of America
Gordon Douglas, Princeton, NJ
John DuMoulin, American College of Physicians-American Society of
    Internal Medicine
Geoffrey Evans, Health Resources and Services Administration
Thomas Fileccia, Department of Defense
John Fontenesi, University of California at San Diego
David Friend, Watson Wyatt Worldwide
Lisa German-Foster, Office of Senator Jack Reed
Geno Germano, Wyeth-Lederle
Barry Gershon, GlaxoSmithKline
Jayne Gilbert, Chiron
Juliana Gonen, Washington Business Group on Health
John Grabenstein, U.S. Army Medical Command
Henry Grabowski, Duke University
Christine Grant, Aventis Pasteur
Robert Gribble, Marshfield Clinic
Claire Hannan, Association of State and Territorial Health Officials
Maxine Hayes, Washington State Health Department
Janet Heinrich, General Accounting Office
Karen Hendricks, American Academy of Pediatrics
Sarah Henning, Marshfield Clinic

Bill Herman, Highsmith Inc.
Susan Hildebrandt, American Association of Family Physicians
Linda Hilson, IMS Health, UK
Phil Hosbach, Aventis Pasteur
William Howell, U.S. Army Medical Research and Materiel Command,
    Fort Detrick, MD
Noreen Hunt, Children's Primary Care Medical Group, San Diego
Hejab Imteyaz, Washington, DC
Jake Jacobs, Capitol Outcomes Research Inc.
Scott Jauch, American College of Physicians-American Society of
    Internal Medicine
Susan Lanza, Health Insurance Association of America
Jo Lecouliard, GlaxoSmithKline
Greg Lehmann, National Business Coalition on Health
Susan Lett, Massachusetts Department of Health
Barbara Levine, Association of State and Territorial Health Officials
Richard Levinson, American Public Health Association
Clement Lewin, Chiron
Joan Mahanes, Centers for Medicare and Medicaid Services
Adel Mahmoud, Merck Vaccine Division
Henri Manasse, American Society of Health System Pharmacists
Eugene Mascolo, Aventis Pasteur
Mark Mathew, Parexel International Corporation
Brian McKenna, Aventis Pasteur
Patrick McLean, GlaxoSmithKline
Suzanne Mercure, National Business Coalition on Health
Jack Meyer, Economic and Social Research Institute
Allen Meyerhoff, Capitol Outcomes Research Inc.
Kent Moore, American Association of Family Physicians
Jessica Mullan, Office of Senator Richard Durbin
Thomas Musco, Health Insurance Association of America
Karen Nielsen, GlaxoSmithKline
Jackie Noyes, American Academy of Pediatrics
Ryan O'Connor, American Medical Group Association
Peter Paradiso, Wyeth-Lederle
Frank Pasquire, General Accounting Office
Jim Pawelski American Academy of Pediatrics
Steve Pearlin, Geisinger Clinic
Dean Perry, Geisinger Clinic
Joe Piascentini, U.S. Department of Labor
Chris Queram, Employer Healthcare Alliance Cooperative
Sarah Radcliff, Pharmaceutical Research and Manufacturers Association
Bob Rehm, American Association of Health Plans

Janice Reichert, Tufts Center for the Study of Drug Development
Robert Shoppe, Marshfield Clinic
David Smith, Texas Tech University
Natalie Smith, California Department of Health Services
Rick Smith, Pharmaceutical Research and Manufacturers Association
Dan Soland, GlaxoSmithKline
Charles Stellar, American Association of Health Plans
Litjen (L.J.) Tan, American Medical Association
Eric Tischler, Aventis Pasteur
Thomas Vernon, Merck Vaccine Division
Dan Walter, American Academy of Pediatrics
Piers Whitehead, VaxGen
Patricia Willis, U.S. Department of Labor
Jillian Woolett, Pharmaceutical Research and Manufacturers Association
Elizabeth (Bitsy) York, GlaxoSmithKline
Herbert Young, American Association of Family Physicians
Barbara Zake, Geisinger Clinic
Jennifer Zavolinsky, American Association of Health Plans
Thomas Zink, GlaxoSmithKline

Appendix C

Survey of State
Vaccine Finance Practices

In 2001, the IOM Committee on the Evaluation of Vaccine Purchase Financing in the United States commissioned a survey from Dr. Gary Freed and his colleagues at the Division of General Pediatrics, University of Michigan. The purpose of this survey was to describe how state health departments finance, purchase, and distribute vaccines; address vaccine shortages; regulate immunization insurance benefits; and allocate scarce resources among vaccine purchase, delivery, and infrastructure investment. This survey was a follow-up to a prior survey of state immunization program practices regarding the scope, structure, financing, and operation of state immunization efforts, conducted by Dr. Freed for an earlier IOM committee (Freed et al., 2000).

The University of Michigan team contacted immunization program managers and project directors of the 50 states and the District of Columbia. Interviews were conducted via telephone and mail during the summer of 2002 and were completed by 48 states. The CDC National Immunization Program provided the names of immunization program managers and project directors in each state, and the IOM sent each a cover letter explaining the nature of the survey interview. CDC also provided state-level background information and documentation, such as copies of grant awards and site visit data. Topics addressed in the interviews included the following:

- Breakdown of funds from VFC, Section 317, state, and any other resources used for vaccine purchase overall

- Changes to the current system of vaccine financing or any new vaccine financing strategies
- Estimates of annual needs for public-sector purchase each year for the child, adolescent, and adult populations
- Adequacy of VFC funding
- Process by which vaccines are ordered from the federal contract
- Purchases of vaccines outside the federal contract
- Distribution to providers and provider choice for publicly purchased vaccines
- Stockpiles and shortages

The report on the survey, *State-Level Perspectives on Vaccine Purchase Financing,* is available through the IOM's public record file.

Appendix D

Overview of Commissioned Papers

The IOM committee commissioned eight background papers as part of the collection of evidence to support this study. The commissioned papers are briefly described below.

1. *Trends In Vaccine Prices, 1992–2002.* Provides a quantitative analysis of vaccine trends using two different data sources, and analyzes the impact of market structure variables on these trends.

Frank Lichtenberg, Graduate School of Business, Columbia University

2. *An Overview of the Market for Vaccines in the United States.* Presents a comprehensive industrial organization analysis of the market for vaccines in the United States, with a focus on production and licensing processes and the mixed public–private market for vaccines.

Richard Arnould and Larry DeBrock, Department of Economics, University of Illinois at Urbana-Champaign

3. *How Insurance Companies and Health Plans Are Planning for New Vaccines.* Through interviews with health plans and state officials, considers how private and public insurance plans make decisions about insurance benefits for vaccine products and provider fees, with a focus on future strategies in light of rising vaccine costs.

Kathy Swartz, School of Public Health, Harvard University

4. *Vaccine Purchase and Distribution: Proposed Changes in Vaccine Supply and Delivery Policies*. Based on a series of interviews with key policy makers, reviews proposals made by industry, government, medical professional organizations, and other stakeholders to fix the current system through a wide range of proposed reforms.

Gerry Fairbrother and Arfana Haidery, New York Academy of Medicine

5. *Setting Prices for New Vaccines (in Advance)*. Presents an economic model for calculating a price for future vaccines in advance as a way to stimulate investment in vaccine development and determine an acceptable price in the absence of a functioning market.

Thomas McGuire, Department of Health Care Policy, Harvard Medical School

6. *Vaccine Policy Perspectives: Market Strategies*. Considers a wide array of strategic options for improving the financing of vaccines through market-based approaches such as price incentives, a voucher system to distribute vaccines, and reduced barriers to global competition in the United States.

Joel Hay and Danielle Zammit, Department of Economics, University of Southern California

7. *Estimating the Need for Publicly Purchased Vaccine for Adults and Children*. Provides estimates of the numbers and characteristics of child and adult populations that require assistance in purchasing vaccines and a description of how such assistance is currently received through state and federal public health and private health care systems.

David Wood, Delmarva Foundation

8. *Diphtheria, Tetanus, and Acellular Pertussis Vaccine (DTaP): A Case Study*. Presents a case study analysis of the DTaP vaccine illustrating the changes in the vaccine market over time; based on structured interviews with regulators, industry executives, and providers.

Amy Fine, Consultant, Washington, DC

Appendix E

Committee and Staff Biographies

FRANK A. SLOAN, Ph.D. (*Chair*) is J. Alexander McMahon Professor of Health Policy and Management, Professor of Economics, and Director, Center for Health Policy, Law & Management, and holds faculty secondary appointments in the Sanford Institute for Public Policy and the Fuqua School of Business at Duke University. Earlier, he served on the faculties of the University of Florida (1971–1976) and Vanderbilt University (1976–1993) and was a research economist at the Rand Corporation (1968–1971). Among his current interests are issues related to aging, including Medicare; health care regulation and competition; prevention of smoking and excess alcohol use; and medical malpractice. He has been a member of IOM since 1982, serving as co-chair of the Committee on the Adequacy of Nurse Staffing (1995–1996) and as a member of the Committee on Veterans Administration Pharmacy Formulary Analysis (1999–2000) and the Committee to Develop a National Research Agenda on Aging (1988–1991). Between January 1990 and December 2002, he served on the IOM Council. He is a co-author of *The Smoking Puzzle: Information, Risk Perceptions, and Choice* (Harvard University Press, 2003).

STEPHEN BERMAN, M.D., is Professor of Pediatrics, Head of the Section of Academic General Pediatrics, and Director of Children's Outcomes Research at the University of Colorado Health Sciences Center and the Children's Hospital Denver. He is also a former President (2000–2001) of the American Academy of Pediatrics (AAP), and previously chaired the AAP Committee on Child Health Financing (1993–1995). Dr. Berman was a member of The National Academies Committee on Acute Respiratory

Infections in Third World Children (1989–1992). He conducts clinical research, teaches, and has written three textbook editions on pediatric algorithms, titled *Pediatric Decision Making.* He is Health Policy Consulting Editor of *Pediatrics.* Dr. Berman has worked in migrant and community health centers and hospital clinics in the United States and South America and has served as an international consultant for the World Health Organization in India, Egypt, and the Philippines and throughout Latin America. Currently he is a practicing pediatrician who provides primary care for children with special health care needs.

DAVID M. CUTLER, Ph.D., is a professor in the department of Economics at the Kennedy School of Government, Harvard University (1991–present). He is also a research associate at the National Bureau of Economic Research, specializing in aging, health care, public economics, and productivity programs. During 1993, Dr. Cutler served as senior staff economist at the Council of Economic Advisers and Director of the National Economic Council. His research examines the impact of medical care on the public sector, the value of medical innovation, and how population health is changing over time. His books include *The Changing Hospital Industry: Comparing Not-for-Profit and For-Profit Hospitals* (University of Chicago Press, 1999) and *Medical Care Productivity and Output* (forthcoming, University of Chicago Press, 2000). He is an editor of the *Journal of Health Economics.* Dr. Cutler recently served on the IOM Committee on Future Research Directions in Behavioral and Social Sciences Research at the National Institutes of Health (NIH) (1999–2001) and the Committee on the NIH Research Priority-Setting Process (1998).

ERIC K. FRANCE, M.D., M.S.P.H., is Chief of Preventive Medicine at Kaiser Permanente Colorado (KPC). He also holds assistant clinical professorships in the Department of Preventive Medicine and Biometrics and the Department of Pediatrics at the Colorado Health Sciences Center. Dr. France served as a liaison member of the Advisory Committee on Immunization Practices (ACIP) and Chair of the Immunization Task Force for the American Association of Health Plans from 1999 to 2002. His research interests include vaccine safety and prevention interventions. He is principal investigator for the KPC Vaccine Safety Datalink project and has focused recently on the safety of the influenza vaccine among children.

WILLIAM J. HALL, M.D., is Paul Fine Professor of Medicine and Director of the Center for Healthy Aging at the University of Rochester School of Medicine and Dentistry. He is the immediate past president of the American College of Physicians–American Society of Internal Medicine (ACP–ASIM), a professional organization representing over 115,000 doctors of internal medicine. Dr. Hall has a long-standing interest in Medicare reform and health policy. His major research interest is in the area of successful aging. He is Director of the Center for Lifetime Wellness, which designs community-based programs in prevention and lifestyle modification for older adults. He serves on a number of national committees addressing issues in geriatrics, including the National Institute for Aging, American Board of Internal Medicine, American Geriatrics Society, John Hartford Foundation, and Donald Reynolds Foundation.

DAVID R. JOHNSON, M.D., M.P.H., is Deputy Director for Public Health and Chief Medical Executive of the Michigan Department of Community Health (1997–present). He also holds an adjunct associate professorship of epidemiology at the University of Michigan School of Public Health and associate clinical professorship in the Department of Pediatrics and Human Development at Michigan State University. Dr. Johnson recently completed a term as a member of the ACIP. While serving on ACIP, he chaired the working group that formulated initial recommendations for the use of conjugate pneumococcal vaccine. He is an executive committee member for the Association of State and Territorial Health Officials and chairs that association's infectious disease policy committee. In 1993, he was awarded a Distinguished Service Award by the Michigan Association of Public Health Physicians.

ALISON KEITH, Ph.D., is an independent consultant who advises nonprofit organizations and businesses on a range of pharmaceutical policy issues. She was previously Director of Economic and Science Policy Analysis at Pfizer, Inc. In this capacity, she directed a wide range of public policy initiatives related to pharmaceutical innovation, direct-to-consumer advertising, health and productivity, pharmaceutical pricing, and Medicare reform. Dr. Keith has also held positions within the Bureau of Economics of the Federal Trade Commission, conducting analyses of consumer protection and antitrust issues. She co-authored the Federal Trade Commission's staff study on *Generic Substitution and Prescription Drug Prices: Economic Effects of State Drug Product Selection Laws*. She has published or reviewed papers for *Managerial and Decision Economics*, *Health Affairs*, the *Journal of Industrial Economics*, the *Journal of Health Economics*, and the *Journal of Law and Economics*. Dr. Keith received a B.A. degree in economics magna cum laude from Carleton College and earned her doctorate in economics from the University of California at Berkeley.

JUNE E. O'NEILL, Ph.D., is Wollman Professor of Economics at the Zicklin School of Business and director of the Center for the Study of Business and Government at Baruch College, City University of New York.

During 1995–1999, she served as director of the Congressional Budget Office. She previously served as director of policy research at the U.S. Commission on Civil Rights (1986–1987), program director and senior research associate at the Urban Institute (1979–1986), and senior economist on the President's Council of Economic Advisors (1971–1976). Dr. O'Neill's published articles and books cover several areas, including wage differentials, welfare, health insurance, tax and budget policy, and social security. She earned a Ph.D. in economics from Columbia University.

MARK V. PAULY, Ph.D., is Bendheim Professor and Chair of the Department of Health Care Systems at Wharton School, University of Pennsylvania, where he has served on the faculty since 1983. Among his recent publications are *Health Benefits at Work: An Economic and Political Analysis of Health Benefits at Work* (AEI Press, 1999) and *Supplying Vaccine: An Economic Analysis of Critical Issues* (IOS Press, 1996). Dr. Pauly served on the IOM Committee on Choice and Managed Care: Furthering the Knowledge Base to Ensure Public Accountability and Information for Informed Purchasing by and on Behalf of Medicare Beneficiaries (1997–1998) and the Committee on Choice and Managed Care: Assuring Public Accountability and Information for Informed Purchasing (1995–1997).

SARA ROSENBAUM, J.D., is Interim Chair of the Department of Health Policy and Hirsh Professor of Health Law and Policy at The George Washington University Medical Center, School of Public Health and Health Services. She also directs the Hirsh Health Law and Policy Program and the Center for Health Services Research and Policy. Professor Rosenbaum has played a major role in the design of federal and state health policy across a wide range of issues. During 1993–1994, she served on the White House Domestic Policy Council and directed the drafting of the Health Security Act for President Clinton. Professor Rosenbaum is co-author of *Law and the American Health Care System* (Foundation Press, 1997) a widely used health law textbook. She also is a recipient of The Robert Wood Johnson Foundation Investigator's Award in Health Policy Research. Professor Rosenbaum has been recognized as one of America's 500 most influential health policy makers.

IRIS R. SHANNON, Ph.D., R.N., is an associate professor in Health Systems Management at Rush University College of Health Sciences (1988–present), where she has also held an associate professorship in the Department of Community Health Nursing (1974–1997). Her research interests are centered on public health nursing and health and social programs that target the poor. She was a member of the IOM Planning Committee on Community Oriented Primary Care (1982). In 1990, she chaired the Committee for the National Center for Nursing Research and Demonstration in Community-based Rural Health Care Models for Minority Populations. Dr. Shannon served as chair of the American Public Health Association's (APHA) Public Health Nursing Section (1988) and is a former President of APHA (1989).

STAFF

ROSEMARY CHALK is study director for the IOM Committee on the Evaluation of Vaccine Purchase Finance in the United States. She has served as a study director or senior program officer for over a dozen studies within the Institute of Medicine and the National Research Council since 1986, including studies on the public health infrastructure for immunization, family violence, child abuse and neglect, research ethics, and education finance. Since 2000, Ms. Chalk has also directed studies on the development of child well-being indicators for the child welfare system at Child Trends in Washington, D.C. She has previously served as a consultant for science and society research projects in Cambridge, MA. She was the program head of the Committee on Scientific Freedom and Responsibility of the American Association for the Advancement of Science from 1976–1986. Ms. Chalk has a B.A. in foreign affairs from the University of Cincinnati.

ROBERT GIFFIN, Ph.D., is senior program officer for the IOM Committee on the Evaluation of Vaccine Purchase Finance in the United States, and is involved in the development of research initiatives in quality and accountability in health care. Before coming to the IOM, he consulted to government, associations, payors, and providers on managed care and finance issues, including the design of state-managed mental health delivery systems, evaluation tools for community health agencies, and new product development for hospitals, managed care organizations, and health care associations. Dr. Giffin teaches graduate economics and strategic management at Georgetown University and the Bethesda Naval Hospital. He previously held senior positions at CIGNA Corporation and the American Association of Health Plans. Dr. Giffin received a Ph.D. in economics from Temple University and a B.A. in American history from Washington University.